P9-DEP-107

OSTEOPOROSIS: ASSESS YOUR RISK

Are you one of the 44 million Americans affected by this disease? The answer may be "yes" if you have:

- An ethnic background that is Caucasian or Asian, though African Americans and Hispanic Americans also have significant risk
- Low estrogen from menopause or a hysterectomy with ovaries removed
- A personal history of fracture after age forty
- A family history of osteoporosis
- A thin or small frame
- A lifelong low intake of calcium
- An inactive lifestyle
- A history of abnormal menstrual periods or anorexia nervosa
- A history of cigarette smoking and/or excessive use of alcohol
- A history of taking corticosteroids, anticonvulsants, and certain other medications
- Diseases such as rheumatoid arthritis or hyperthyroidism
- Low testosterone levels if you are male.

The good news is that you *can* take charge of your health and reduce your risk of bone loss. Find out . . .

WHAT YOUR DOCTOR MAY *NOT* TELL YOU ABOUT OSTEOPOROSIS

WHAT YOUR DOCTOR MAY *NOT* TELL YOU ABOUT OSTEOPOROSIS

Help Prevent—and Even Reverse— the Disease That Burdens Millions of Women

FELICIA COSMAN, M.D.

clinical director, National Osteoporosis Foundation

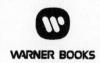

WARNER BOOKS

An AOL Time Warner Company

If you purchase this book without a cover you should be aware that this book may have been stolen property and reported as "unsold and destroyed" to the publisher. In such case neither the author nor the publisher has received any payment for this "stripped book."

This book is not intended as a substitute for medical advice of physicians. The reader should regularly consult a physician in all matters relating to his or her health, and particularly in respect to any symptoms that may require diagnosis or medical attention.

Copyright © 2003 by Felicia Cosman, M.D.
All rights reserved.

The title of the series What Your Doctor May *Not* Tell You about . . . and the related trade dress are trademarks owned by Warner Books, Inc., and may not be used without permission.

Warner Books, Inc., 1271 Avenue of the Americas, New York, NY 10020
Visit our Web site at www.twbookmark.com

 An AOL Time Warner Company

Printed in the United States of America

First Printing: May 2003
10   9   8   7   6   5   4   3   2   1

Library of Congress Cataloging-in-Publication Data
Cosman, Felicia
    What your doctor may not tell you about osteoporosis : help prevent and even reverse the disease that burdens millions of women / Felicia Cosman.
        p. cm.
    Includes index.
    ISBN 0-446-67903-8
    1. Osteoporosis—Popular works. 2. Osteoporosis in women—Popular works. I. Title.

RC931.O73 C67 2003
616.7'16—dc21   2002193356

Cover design by Diane Luger
Book design by Charles A. Sutherland

This book is dedicated to the memory of my beloved parents, Sylvia Rose Cosman (1924–1988) and Cantor Ian Cosman (1909–1990). They had endless love, generosity, devotion, warmth, intelligence, strength, and zest for life. I still miss them every single day of my life.

Acknowledgments

Most major endeavors, such as writing this book, cannot be achieved without the love and support of family. For this, I thank my wonderful husband, Dr. Neville Clynes, and three beautiful children, Sasha, Arielle, and Matthew; my brothers, Jeffrey and Maury; brothers-in-law, Darius, Raphael, and Lawrence; my sisters-in-law, Jacqueline, Carol, and Joan; my mother-in-law, Renate; father-in-law, Manfred; my more extended family, especially my cousin Shae and his family, and my surviving as well as my deceased aunts and uncles and other cousins and close friends (especially Ron and Hagit Mass), all of whom have influenced my life.

I'd also like to thank my boss, colleague, and very good friend, Dr. Robert Lindsay: a true pioneer in the field of women's health, the first to establish conclusively the role of estrogen therapy in maintenance of bone health in women after menopause; my very good friend and colleague, epidemiologist Dr. Jeri Nieves, a stalwart force in my life and a daily bouncing board for ideas, both professional and personal; and my many colleagues at Helen Hayes Hospital with whom I have worked closely over the years, especially Shari, Michelle, David, Sandra, Adrianne, Lillian, Joann, Nancy, Susan, Marsha, Patricia, Rosemarie, Judy, Michael, Mercedes, and Terri.

My deep appreciation also goes to colleagues outside Helen Hayes Hospital, particularly Dr. Steve Cummings, a brilliant clinical research scientist and a tremendously kind and supportive mentor; my colleagues and friends at Columbia (New York Presbyterian Hospital) who helped get me started, especially Dr. Ethel Siris and Dr. John Bilezikian; and my friends in the pharmaceutical industry, particularly Sharon Scurato.

I thank and acknowledge the National Osteoporosis Foundation, an advocacy organization devoted to education, research, and care of people with osteoporosis. This dedicated, sensitive, and intelligent group of people has increased awareness of osteoporosis dramatically and has influenced the lives of many people suffering from or at significant risk of developing the disease.

My sincere gratitude goes to all the women and men who have participated in clinical research protocols at Helen Hayes Hospital and throughout the world. Medical treatments could not advance without these courageous and generous individuals.

I also wish to thank my patients for sharing their lives with me. It has provided me enormous satisfaction getting to know them over the years, advising them about osteoporosis and other health issues and sharing with them the triumphs and tragedies of their lives and the lives of their families. I hope I have helped some of them cope better, and enjoy their lives more.

Contents

Acknowledgments   vii
Introduction   xi

PART I: UNDERSTANDING OSTEOPOROSIS   1

CHAPTER 1. My Personal Journey   3
CHAPTER 2. What Is Osteoporosis?   9
CHAPTER 3. The Architecture of a Disease   22

PART II: PREVENTING AND SLOWING THE
            EFFECTS OF OSTEOPOROSIS   35

CHAPTER 4. Prevention: The Universal Message   37
CHAPTER 5. Prevention Step One: Reducing Risk
            Factors   40
CHAPTER 6. Prevention Step Two: Nutrition   49
CHAPTER 7. Prevention Step Three: Exercise   72
CHAPTER 8. Prevention Step Four: Supplements and
            Vitamins?   89

PART III: DIAGNOSING OSTEOPOROSIS   101

CHAPTER 9. Are You at Risk?   103

CHAPTER 10. Getting Tested: Measuring and
　　　　　　Reporting Bone Mass　　　　　　　112
CHAPTER 11. Blood and Urine Tests and Radiologic
　　　　　　Procedures　　　　　　　　　　　129

PART IV: MEDICATION AND TREATMENT　　　141

CHAPTER 12. Fracture Care and Rehabilitation　　143
CHAPTER 13. Medication for Osteoporosis in Women　158
CHAPTER 14. Estrogen or Hormone Therapy　　　165
CHAPTER 15. Selective Estrogen Receptor Modulators　182
CHAPTER 16. Calcitonin　　　　　　　　　　193
CHAPTER 17. Bisphosphonates　　　　　　　200
CHAPTER 18. Parathyroid Hormone　　　　　214
CHAPTER 19. Non-FDA-Approved Treatments　　226
CHAPTER 20. Monitoring Treatment　　　　　235

PART V: SPECIAL CASES　　　　　　　　　241

Chapter 21. Men　　　　　　　　　　　　243
Chapter 22. The Premenopausal Woman　　　249
Chapter 23. Osteoporosis Associated with Steroids　256

Afterword: The Future　　　　　　　　　　263

Appendix A: Interpreting Medical Evidence　　265

Appendix B: Web Sites with Good Information about
　　　　　　Osteoporosis　　　　　　　　　277

Introduction

The facts:

Osteoporosis and low bone mass are currently estimated to be a major public health threat for almost forty-four million U.S. women and men aged fifty and over. One in two Caucasian and Asian women eventually suffer from the disease; the rate is one in five for black women. A woman's risk of hip fracture is equal to her combined risk of breast, uterine, and ovarian cancer. As the baby boomer generation ages in the next few decades, the economic and societal impact of hip fracture due to osteoporosis will only increase. Currently, we spend approximately fourteen billion dollars per year on osteoporosis-related fractures and their consequences. It is estimated that in the next two decades, by the year 2020, this number will more than double, with estimated costs of thirty billion per year (statistics from the National Osteoporosis Foundation).

Due to these shocking statistics, there is a public health mandate to try to reduce the occurrence of the disease; no national medical system will be able to comfortably absorb this cost. This has resulted in a stimulation of federally funded research, which has dramatically advanced our understanding of the mechanisms of disease and management, and has laid the groundwork for the development of effective therapies for osteoporosis.

This book is intended to fill in the holes left by visits with doctors who have limited time to educate their patients. The current medical system in the United States is not designed to allow for the hours necessary to discuss osteoporosis: its impact on patients, preventive measures, how to diagnose it, and how to determine the appropriate treatment for each individual patient.

All chronic diseases require substantial patient education, because people have to live with them for a long time. This is certainly true of osteoporosis, as well as high blood pressure, high blood cholesterol, and the possible outcomes of stroke and heart attack or heart failure. It is also true, to some extent, of cancer, especially when it comes to prevention and treatment, where nutritional factors and lifestyle may play a role. The more people know about the disease, the more empowered they will be to live with it well and reduce its burden.

Of course, the pharmaceutical industry is driven by potential profits from the aging population at risk of osteoporosis. This is very fortunate, since the mutual needs of society as a whole and the pharmaceutical industry have resulted in the osteoporosis field moving very rapidly. On average, new drugs have come out almost yearly since 1995, with the introduction of nasal calcitonin, alendronate, raloxifene, risedronate, and, most recently, parathyroid hormone. Many more therapeutic agents are also on the horizon or in clinical or laboratory testing. Thankfully, research and drug development programs have resulted in a dramatic improvement in our ability to reduce the impact of this often disfiguring, painful, and disabling disease.

I strongly believe that if there are no data supporting the effectiveness and safety of a medication for a specific purpose, then there is no reason to take it. This relates not only to prescription medications, but also to the so-called nutritional supplements and vitamins. The information presented in this book is based on a rational interpretation of scientific and medical evidence. One of the appendices of this book explains the different types of medical evidence that we consider when evaluating the effectiveness of a medical therapy and discusses the rating of evidence and its rationale. Where there is little available information, I will try to make it clear and will provide what I think are reasonable recommendations based on my fifteen years of experience caring for patients with osteoporosis and people trying to prevent it.

HOW TO USE THIS BOOK

The first section of the book describes the disease and some of its causes, and discusses its impact on the lives of people who suffer from it. In the second section, the steps toward prevention of osteoporosis are highlighted, including lifestyle changes, nutrition, and exercise. The third section concentrates on how to determine your risk of osteoporosis and discusses diagnosis of the disease, with particular attention to the meaning and reporting of bone mass measurements and the distinction between osteoporosis and osteopenia. It also briefly talks about some of the other tests that would be recommended in certain circumstances for some patients. In the fourth section, all the medical and nonmedical treatments for osteoporosis are discussed. Since osteoporosis is most common in postmenopausal women, the majority of the book is about this type of osteoporosis, but the final section of the book considers other patients—men, premenopausal women, and patients receiving steroid treatments. Each chapter is capped by a "Bare Bones" of what you need to know—a summary of key points and advice.

My goals in writing this book are to empower patients with the tools they need to help prevent disease and enable them to go to their doctors with questions and requests. Hopefully you will find in these pages the knowledge necessary to help you or your loved ones participate in decision making with doctors, allay your fears, and alleviate your suffering.

Part I

UNDERSTANDING OSTEOPOROSIS

Chapter 1

My Personal Journey

I first considered having a bone density test when I turned forty a few years ago, but not because I was overly concerned about osteoporosis, ironically. I had decided I was done with childbearing after having three perfectly healthy, wonderful children. I had always thought that I should strongly consider having my ovaries removed preventively, since my mother succumbed to an incredibly virulent form of ovarian cancer in the prime of her life. In addition to my family history, one of the important components of this decision was determining my risk of osteoporosis. As an osteoporosis specialist, I had ready access to bone density testing—the only way to accurately determine osteoporosis risk—but I had never had the test done because I was always either pregnant, nursing, or anticipating becoming pregnant.

Even though I'd been meaning to get the bone density test, what directly precipitated my going in was that a good friend of a similar age was having a screening colonoscopy (her father had died from colon cancer). We had also both had our first mammograms about a year or two earlier. This seemed like a good time to round out the medical picture.

I didn't anticipate anything dramatic in my bone density measurement results. My guess was that I would be close to average. I was always of average size, had regular menstrual periods, no significant smoking history, no excessive alcohol intake, good basic nutrition, and fairly regular exercise. I have always been strong and healthy. Nothing to worry about.

How wrong I was! It turned out that my spine bone mass was in the lower 1 percent for my age. That meant I had full-blown osteoporosis, with a spinal bone mass T-Score of –2.7 (see chapter 10). Comparing my age-matched results (Z-Score) to those of a majority of my patients, my bone mass was worse than almost all of them. Of course, I repeated the test a few times; it just couldn't be right, but all the results came out very similarly. I was numb with the fear that my back would crumble, I would become deformed and disabled, lose six inches of height, and suffer from chronic back pain, when just ten minutes earlier I'd been a healthy young woman with an absolutely fantastic life.

I shared my bad news with everyone—especially my friends and colleagues at work. We joke now about how I mentioned my bone mass every single day at our daily lunch for at least a year. Every time I came down from the outpatient department at my hospital after seeing patients, I mentioned that my bone mass was far worse than anyone I had seen that day. I had some blood and urine tests done to try to exclude any possible underlying diseases that might cause such a low bone mass (see chapter 11). These tests didn't reveal much of anything. In the days when I first began working in the osteoporosis field, I would have definitely recommended a bone biopsy in a person such as myself. Bone biopsies were occasionally done in patients with particularly low bone mass for their age to help exclude other diseases and to try to gauge the underlying bone turnover rate. Doctors are not doing many of these anymore, except for research purposes. Blood and urine tests have largely taken over for both of these purposes.

I remembered that my mother had had some compression fractures of the spine, seen on X ray, when she was having tests done for the abdominal discomfort that ended up being ovarian cancer. At the time, it was just an incidental finding, of little importance compared to her primary disease. My brother said she often had backaches, though she never complained of any serious back pain and never sought medical advice. She stoically worked through any pains or illnesses. She did have a bit of a stooped posture and had lost some height from her peak at five feet, eight inches. This was 1987, a time when there was little discussion about osteoporosis and bone density tests were not yet standard medical practice. Little was known about prevention or treatment, so I put this out of my mind. However, there is no doubt that having a family history such as mine puts you at higher risk for having the disease yourself. In fact, it may be one of the most important factors. In assessing your risk of osteoporosis, you must be familiar with the medical history of your parents and grandparents (see chapter 9). Many people think that if you have osteoporosis, it always means that you've lost a lot of bone. In fact, you might just have been born with very low bone mass.

I'd like to be able to say that I started taking a pill and now everything's fine. That may be the case in a few years, but at the time, because I was so young and still premenopausal, there was very little that I could do about my discovery. In terms of general preventive measures, I had already begun taking calcium supplements and trying to modify my diet to contain enough total calcium. I had already embarked on an exercise program, including both jogging and strength training. I didn't smoke or consume excessive alcohol. I wasn't on any medication that could be altered. My periods were totally regular. And since there weren't (and still aren't) medications proven safe or effective—or approved by the Food and Drug Administration (FDA)—for the treatment of otherwise healthy premenopausal women, I couldn't take any kind of miracle pill. With one exception (PTH or parathyroid hormone), the medications currently on the market work by returning the bone turnover process from the accelerated levels seen in postmenopausal women to the normal levels of premenopausal women. The drugs simply slow down the bone loss process. If bone turnover levels are in the normal premenopausal range to begin with, there is less of a potential effect that these medications could have on bone metabolism. In general, premenopausal women manifest little total skeletal bone loss until they reach the perimenopausal phase of life. So it's likely that these drugs wouldn't work so well in a healthy premenopausal woman.

The one possibility open to me was to try the oral contraceptive pill. There had been a few studies suggesting that women who took the pill had higher bone mass than women who did not. I also thought it might be wise to try the pill for other reasons—namely, its use in premenopausal women has been linked to a reduction in risk of ovarian cancer. I thought I could take care of two problems with one pill, but when I tried a few different preparations, they all left me nauseated and lethargic. I simply couldn't tolerate them. Furthermore, I was unlucky enough to require a breast biopsy about a year after all of this, and the open issue about whether oral contraceptive use might be associated with a small increase in the risk of breast cancer made me feel less sure of the option. Finally, the potentially positive bone effects of the pill were not, and are still not, proven.

So I was a healthy forty-year-old woman with osteoporosis and nothing to do except follow the preventive measures that all of us should be practicing anyway! It was obvious to me that when I reached menopause, I would need some type of medication, and probably should continue taking one for the rest of my life. There was no evidence that anything active was going on in my skeleton; it was likely that I happened to have been born with an extremely low bone mass, largely due to genetic factors. But I felt fine! Osteoporosis is a symptomless condition for many years or even decades. The major challenge at that point was to work on my psychology. Did it make sense to limit my activity to prevent fractures? No way. Not surprisingly, I had never had a fracture—fractures from osteoporosis are exceedingly rare in premenopausal women, even with low bone mass. I simply needed to forget about this until the time when my periods became irregular and continue doing what I was doing anyway. Of course, this was a bit hard to do considering that I was confronted daily with the often devastating consequences of the disease. Additionally, there is not a single day of my professional life that I don't look at one or more bone density test results.

Ultimately, this is why I am opposed to routine bone density screening in premenopausal women. (This does not mean that women with specific diseases or on certain medications should not be tested or treated. In otherwise healthy women, however, it should not be routinely done.) Many young women come to see me after a bone density test with results substantially higher than those I had. Some of them have been told they have severe "bone loss" and have already been put on medicines without proven efficacy or safety in their age group. Some of these women may be having children in the near future, and the impact of these drugs on fetal development is unknown. I am extremely sympathetic to these young women, since I know the fear they have to face. It is a true psychological challenge; I don't think that finding out about osteoporosis at an early age, when there's nothing you can do about it, is necessary or even healthy. Some people would argue that getting a test may help younger women stick with good preventive measures, but there is little evidence to support this argument, and it is hard to justify the cost of these tests in a medical system already overburdened with expenditures.

That said, it's imperative to find out about your osteoporosis risk at the time of menopause, or at the latest by the age of sixty to sixty-five. It would be irresponsible to be ignorant of a diagnosis for which treatment can dramatically modify the course of the disease. This is why I stress throughout the book that we should concentrate our diagnostic and treatment efforts on older individuals, in whom the probability of osteoporosis is much higher, the frequency of fracture occurrence is much higher, and the effectiveness of treatment has been tested and proven.

The fear and worry that I've personally experienced in my battle against osteoporosis have helped me generate a unique professional perspective and empathy for my patients. Humor, perspective, and the certain knowledge that there will be medications available when I need them are what help me cope with my condition. There is also comfort in knowing that I am doing everything I can at this stage, and will continue to do so in the future, to prevent myself from suffering from the consequences of osteoporosis. I fervently hope that readers of this book will come away with similar knowledge and comfort.

Chapter 2

~

What Is Osteoporosis?

A sixty-five-year-old woman is overjoyed, looking for a beautiful outfit to wear to her son's wedding. She notices a hump on her upper back and realizes that she has lost several inches in height. None of the clothes look right on her. All the jackets seem to be pulling up in the back. Even though she is very slim, she feels that her belly is sticking out. She leaves the store sad and disgusted.

At the beginning of springtime, a fifty-two-year-old woman goes to open a window to ventilate her home and suddenly gets a severe sharp stabbing pain in the middle of her back that takes her breath away. She is taken to the hospital, where an X ray shows that she has broken her back.

A seventy-eight-year-old man gets up from bed to go to the bathroom, but his foot gets tangled in the covers and he falls on his side. He has so much pain in his hip and groin area that he can't stand up. It takes an hour to crawl to a phone, but he manages to get 911. After the ambulance ride, an

X ray in the emergency room confirms that he has broken his hip, and the orthopedist on call tells him he will need surgery. He recovers from the surgery but cannot walk up or down stairs, making it impossible to go back to his home. Instead, he is sent to a nursing home.

While going out food shopping, a totally healthy fifty-six-year-old woman slips on a patch of ice on her driveway. She lands with her hands forward and breaks her wrist. A hard cast is required for six weeks to fix the fracture, and she experiences pain throughout this time. It is impossible to cook the huge Christmas dinner that her family is accustomed to.

After a two-week trip helping her daughter with her newborn first baby, a sixty-two-year-old woman gets a bear hug from her husband and feels severe pain in her side. By the next day the pain has not abated, so she goes to her doctor, who orders an X ray of the ribs on the side. The X ray shows she has broken her rib.

An eighty-one-year-old woman has had severe back pain for years. She is practically housebound by pain and by a severe arching deformity of her back that makes it very difficult for her to walk. After being visited by a grandchild who has a cold, she also develops a cold. This is followed by a bad cough ultimately diagnosed as postviral pneumonia. Because of her severe thorax deformity, caused by multiple vertebral compression fractures, she has trouble clearing her secretions, cannot recover from a serious pneumonia, and never makes it out of the hospital.

These are just some of the many faces of osteoporosis.

In this chapter, I'll define osteoporosis, discuss how common it is, and detail the symptoms and impact of the disease, concentrating on the consequences of vertebral and hip fractures, the two most devastating osteoporosis-related fractures.

WHAT IS OSTEOPOROSIS?

Osteoporosis is a generalized disorder of the skeleton in which the amount of bone tissue is reduced and the microscopic structure or architecture of bone is abnormal. Both the abnormal quantity and quality of the bone make it weak and susceptible to breaking given even minimal amounts of trauma. The result of osteoporosis can be viewed as skeletal failure, similar to the development of heart failure after years of uncontrolled high blood pressure. There is no documented evidence that bone loss or reduced bone tissue itself, in the absence of a fracture, is associated with pain or any other symptoms. This means that there are no symptoms of osteoporosis per se, only the consequences: fractures and associated chronic pain, deformity, and disability.

It is important to make the distinction between osteoporosis and osteoarthritis. Often people tell me upon first meeting that they have "osteo." My question is always, "Osteo what?" Osteoporosis is a disorder in which the bones become weak and susceptible to fracturing. Osteoarthritis affects the spaces between the bones, or joint spaces, which contain cartilage, other connective tissue, and shock-absorbing fluid. The joint becomes swollen, inflamed, and deformed, the cartilage is eroded, and bone spurs (small pieces of bone tissue outside the normal confines of the bone) may grow. The causes and treatments of osteoarthritis are very different from those of osteoporosis—although many people suffer from both diseases. Sometimes arthritis can be the result of fractures or fracture healing, which can both produce abnormal forces across the joint.

HOW COMMON IS OSTEOPOROSIS?

Almost one in every two Caucasian women will suffer an osteoporosis-related fracture at some point in her lifetime. The corresponding number of Caucasian men is one in four. Black women have a risk that is similar to that of white men, and black men are at lower, though still substantial, risk. The greater risk in women versus men is related to smaller body size, smaller bone size, lower bone mass at its peak (see below), and greater loss of bone in midlife due to the menopause. The early postmenopausal years are associated with a specific increased risk for the occurrence of wrist and vertebral fractures. While wrist fracture frequency does not increase further as women get older, almost all other osteoporosis-related fractures continue to increase in occurrence with advancing age.

VERTEBRAL FRACTURES

Vertebral fractures occur in the part of the bone called the vertebral body. This is normally a cube-shaped piece of bone that projects forward toward the belly from the spinal processes that you feel when you run your hand along the back (see figure 2-1). When fractured, the bone actually compresses in on itself, unable to sustain the body's weight. Imagine the top half of a glass cube shattering, with the shards of glass falling into the bottom section of the cube. The bone actually shatters and falls in on itself. This type of fracture is very distinct from a fracture in a long bone such as the arm or leg. Furthermore, these fractures

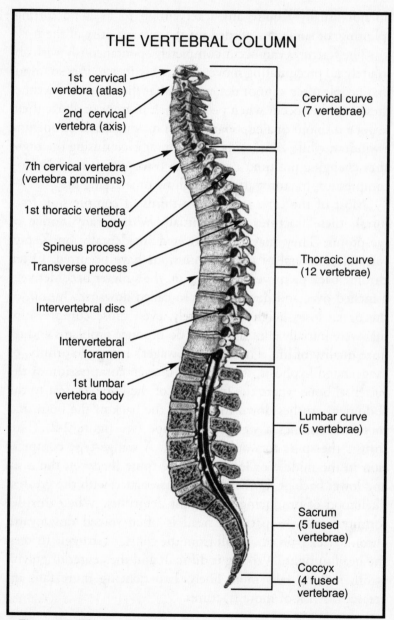

THE VERTEBRAL COLUMN

1st cervical
vertebra (atlas)

2nd cervical
vertebra (axis)

Cervical curve
(7 vertebrae)

7th cervical vertebra
(vertebra prominens)

1st thoracic vertebra
body

Spineus process

Transverse process

Thoracic curve
(12 vertebrae)

Intervertebral disc

Intervertebral
foramen

1st lumbar
vertebra body

Lumbar curve
(5 vertebrae)

Sacrum
(5 fused
vertebrae)

Coccyx
(4 fused
vertebrae)

Figure 2-1: The vertebral column, lateral view.

do not usually require any intervention to heal; no casting, splinting, or surgery is needed for the vast majority of them.

The fractures can occur completely spontaneously with absolutely no precipitating movements, or with activities so minor that people often cannot remember what they were. Sometimes these fractures occur when people reach in front or above them to get a dish out of a cupboard, when making a bed or opening a window, while vacuuming the floor, or even during the night after changing position. People with osteoporosis may develop compression fractures after a coughing or sneezing fit.

Most of the time (about two-thirds of compression fractures), these fractures occur initially without any notice or symptoms. They may be discovered incidentally on X rays years after several of the compressions have occurred. Often chronic back pain eventually sets in, the sufferer becomes very hunched over and develops the so-called dowager's hump, or she or he loses height. Ultimately, even those compressions that were initially clinically silent do produce problems and reduce quality of life. The classic dowager's hump deformity, or exaggerated kyphosis, is due to an uneven compression of the vertebral bone where the front part of the bone, closest to the abdomen, crushes down more than the back of the bone and therefore assumes a wedge-type shape (see figure 2-2). This thrusts the spine forward over itself. A wedge-type compression in the middle or lower thoracic spine (between the neck and lower back or lumbar spine) is associated with the greatest likelihood of producing significant deformity. When this deformity occurs, a patient's head is often forced downward; chronic neck pain can result from the constant struggle to keep the head upright. Walking is difficult and the center of gravity is off, making falls more likely. Experiencing more falls increases the risk of more fractures.

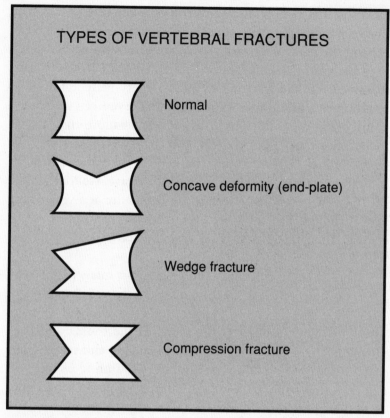

Figure 2-2: Osteoporotic fracture results in a change in the shape of the vertebral body. The shapes here are listed in order of increasing severity from top to bottom.

Since the bone itself loses height during compression, there is often height loss that can be very dramatic. An important manifestation of the loss of height in the thorax is restricted breathing, with an inability to fully expand the chest cavity, resulting in shortness of breath upon limited activity. This is probably one of the reasons why multiple vertebral fractures are associated with an increased risk of premature death, often due to pneumonias and other lung problems. It is difficult to expand the chest fully and to clear secretions normally.

One young male patient of mine, whom I met very early in my career, had fractures of almost every vertebral bone of the thoracic and lumbar spine (a total of seventeen vertebrae). Consequently, he suffered a height loss of more than twelve inches, from a peak of six feet, two inches, to just under five feet, one inch. Unfortunately, we had very few therapeutic alternatives available at that time, and this brave, wonderful man died of complications related to a hip fracture at a very young age. Although he had a very rare and severe form of osteoporosis, the principles that his case illustrates apply to others with less severe cases.

In addition to deformity and height loss, many people who have multiple vertebral fractures also experience chronic back pain. This may be due to the abnormal stretching of muscles, ligaments, and tendons as the shape of the thorax and back changes. This pain is very difficult to control and may require intermittent resting in bed or a supine position to be relieved. On the other hand, patients can often keep going for an hour or two with their usual activities after resting the muscles and other connective tissues by lying down for just fifteen minutes.

Once a certain number of these compressions have occurred, the heights of the lower thorax and/or upper abdomen are reduced such that the few inches of space that normally exist between the lower rib cage and the iliac crests (protruding hip bones) are obliterated (see figure 2-3). This results in chronic pain around the flank area, often relieved only when patients are lying down on their backs.

Additionally, with loss of height in the abdominal cavity, the abdomen is often distended. The contents of the abdominal cavity (all the organs, including the liver, stomach, and intestines) need a certain volume of space, and if the height dimension is reduced they push outward, thereby increasing the depth or girth around the middle. Thus, even very thin women appear to have a protuberant abdomen. Due to the cramped space, there is often an inability to eat a full meal, abdominal discomfort, and constipation and excess gas. With all these chronic symptoms, patients can become depressed and socially isolated.

We don't really understand why some people feel absolutely no symptoms and others experience excruciating pain from these fractures (only about one-third of the time). Those who do have acute symptoms from a fracture often feel a sharp, stabbing-type pain in the back at the point where the fracture occurs. Sometimes the pain can irritate nerve roots and produce pain that radiates around the side of the thorax or abdomen. The sharp pain may be accompanied by muscle spasms, which catch a person's breath. Associated with the fracture, there may be severe constipation related to temporary paralysis of the surrounding intestine.

There are many causes of back pain, including degenerative disk disease (or herniated disks), muscle strain, ligament sprain, osteoarthritis, and others, in addition to osteoporosis with vertebral compressions. So obviously, these other entities need to be excluded by a good doctor evaluating the symptoms. Several of these conditions can coexist. Anyone diagnosed with a vertebral fracture should have a bone density test to confirm the diagnosis of osteoporosis (see chapter 10). Likewise, people who have osteoporosis and back pain should have an X ray to make sure that they don't have vertebral fractures.

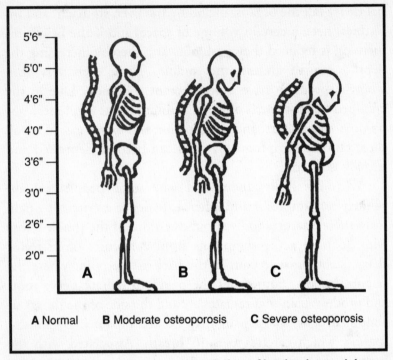

Figure 2-3: Consequences of osteoporosis: loss of height, dowager's hump, change of shape in trunk, and ribs sitting on top of hip bones.

HIP FRACTURES

By far, the fracture that causes the most misery in osteoporosis is the hip fracture. These fractures occur at the top of the thigh bone or femur. They almost always occur in a fall, usually from standing height. They increase dramatically in frequency in women after age sixty-five and in men after age seventy, with progressive increases in risk with advancing age. Hip fractures are accompanied by severe pain in the groin, buttock, or hip, and almost always render the victim unable to stand or walk. Victims are usually taken by ambulance to the emergency room of the nearest hospital and, once medically stabilized, are taken to surgery to fix the fracture. Hip fractures are so serious that for people to walk again, surgical fixation must almost always be done.

Because the hip fracture requires surgical repair, there are surgical complications. Infections, bleeding, and blood clots are all possible. The risk of dying in the year following the fracture is 15 to 20 percent higher than in a group of individuals of the same age with no hip fracture. Many patients will need rehabilitation to make any reasonable recovery. Hip fractures are frequently one of the ways in which healthy older people begin to suffer major disability. Many hip fracture victims (25 percent) must go to a nursing home, one of the biggest fears of the elderly. There are multiple reasons for this—they may not recover enough mobility because of pain or slow healing of the fracture; they may be specifically told not to put much weight on the leg during the first few weeks of healing (because of the type of fracture repair), making it difficult to climb and descend stairs in their homes; they may suffer mental decline related to the trauma of the surgery or its aftermath; or they may suffer medical complications from the hip fracture and added functional limitations. Many of the victims who can go home after surgical repair require assistance at home to accomplish tasks that were previously simple: bathing, getting to the toilet, dressing, grooming, cooking, shopping, and cleaning house. Many women and men who suffer hip fractures need canes or walkers to walk safely. Only about 15 percent of people regain the same independence that they had prior to the occurrence of the fracture.

OTHER FRACTURES

I thought I had seen it all in the arena of osteoporosis until a patient with an extremely severe case came to see me a few weeks ago. Apparently about a year earlier, she had been sitting having Thanksgiving dinner with her family and felt her neck fall forward. She sort of held it up with her hands and somehow managed to survive the car ride home from Connecticut to New York. She fell asleep but the following day, she awoke with severe neck pain and saw her primary doctor. Nothing was seen initially but a few days later, when she returned to the doctor with continued pain and neck weakness, she was told she'd broken her neck. She had major surgery to stabilize several vertebrae, and although she is not pain-free right now and wears a brace to keep her head propped up, at least she did not suffer any neurologic problems such as a torn spinal cord in the neck. This is an exceedingly rare complication of osteoporosis, and probably occurred in part as a result of severe deformity—the neck being thrust dramatically forward from severe osteoporosis.

A fracture of any bone can occur in osteoporosis and cause temporary pain and disability, if not permanent disability or death. Rib fractures often occur upon coughing, sneezing, banging into something, or engaging in a tight hug. Pelvic fractures can occur in a fall or sometimes spontaneously. Rib and pelvic breaks rarely require any surgery, casting, or splinting. They heal with rest. Wrist fractures are a common manifestation of osteoporosis. These usually respond to casting but sometimes require surgical repair.

Many people, as they relate their histories, tell me that they fractured because they fell. Most people don't realize that the same fall in a younger, healthier person with a better bone mass would most likely not have resulted in a fracture. In fact, most adulthood fractures that occur in the absence of a major trauma, such as a motor vehicle accident, a bungee-jumping accident—are attributable, at least to some degree, to osteoporosis.

THE BARE BONES

- Osteoporosis produces weakening of the bones, making them susceptible to breaking or fracturing with little trauma.
- Almost half of all white women and a quarter of all white men will experience an osteoporosis-related fracture at some point in their lifetimes. Hispanics have a risk similar to that of Caucasians; Asians have slightly lower risk. Black women and men are at lower, but still substantial, risk.
- Hip and spine fractures have the most devastating consequences in osteoporosis, but fractures of any bone can occur.
- Although spine fractures can produce severe sudden back pain, many of these fractures occur without notice at the time of the event. Ultimately they often lead to height loss, deformity, chronic pain, difficulty breathing, and abdominal distension and pain.
- Hip fractures are associated with a high rate of death over the first year following the fracture and frequently produce loss of independence and permanent disability. They are the most common diagnosis for patients entering nursing homes.

Chapter 3

The Architecture of a Disease

For the most part, *osteoporosis* can be defined as a disease in which bone mass is reduced enough to substantially increase the risk of fracture. Bone mass at any point is a function of all the beneficial and detrimental things that have occurred prior to the measurement. It is useful to understand how the skeleton might end up in a compromised state by separately evaluating the two major stages of changes in bone mass: the amount of bone gain (or acquisition of peak bone mass) and the subsequent amount of bone loss (see figure 3-1). At any adult age, the measured bone mass level is the result of the amount of bone attained at peak age (peak bone mass) minus the amount of bone lost. Unless bone mass has been measured during young adulthood, however, it is impossible to actually know how much bone has been lost by later adulthood. In fact, it is a common misinterpretation of bone mass measurement for physicians to tell patients that they have lost tremendous amounts of bone on the basis of a single measurement. Although we cannot actually measure the amount of bone loss, we know the factors that can influence it. This chapter will review the factors known to be important to both gaining bone (and achieving the highest possible peak bone mass) and preventing bone loss, as well as touching on the bone quality factors also known to be important in increasing or decreasing the risk of fracture.

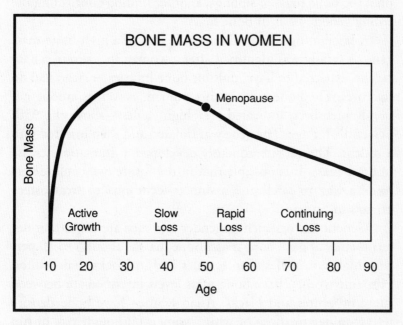

Figure 3-1: Peak bone mass is achieved by age twenty-five, plateaus between ages thirty and forty, and undergoes a dramatic reduction around the time of menopause.

PEAK BONE MASS

Peak bone mass, the highest amount of bone that a person achieves in life, usually occurs by age twenty-five. The bone that can be achieved at this stage is predetermined by an individual's genetic makeup. There are probably several genes involved, and the tendency to have a low bone mass or osteoporosis can be transmitted through either the mother's or the father's family, as shown by bone mass studies of mothers and daughters as well as fathers and daughters. Furthermore, identical twins have bone mass measurements much more similar than the bone mass of siblings, another finding confirming the strong genetic basis of bone mass.

A fascinating recent discovery is that of a high-bone-mass gene. A family was identified after a woman in a severe car accident, expected to have multiple bone injuries, instead had no fractures. The bone mass in this woman, as well as among her family members, indicated very high values—above the 95th percentile for age. The gene was isolated and then injected into a rodent. The rat subsequently developed a dramatic increase in bone mass. It is possible that in the future, we could determine a way to safely use a similar technique to treat osteoporosis in humans.

Genetic factors such as gender and race are important determinants of peak bone mass. Bone mass is about 5 to 10 percent higher in males than females and in blacks than whites. Hispanic women have bone mass levels intermediate between those of whites and blacks. Asian women have bone density levels similar to those of white women (although risk of hip fracture is slightly lower in Asians than Caucasians due to racial differences in shape, length, and geometry of the hip). There are some differences in physiology between blacks and whites with respect to bone turnover and the amount of calcium excretion in the urine, as well as body and bone size and body composition, but the full explanation for racial differences in bone mass is not known. Gender differences in levels of bone mass at the peak are also in part related to bone and body size differences.

Optimal lifestyle factors such as good overall nutrition with adequate calcium intake and regular physical activity can help a young person achieve her or his genetically predetermined bone mass. Having regular menstrual periods is also necessary for a young woman to achieve her genetic potential for peak bone mass. Girls or young women who have anorexia nervosa or exercise excessively may not attain the peak mass they should have (based on their genetic endowment), in part because of irregular or absent menstrual periods, reflecting a lower level of overall estrogen production. Smoking and excessive alcohol consumption might negatively affect the bone mass achieved at peak. Young children who have certain diseases such as diabetes mellitus or rheumatoid arthritis may also be unable to achieve their genetically determined peak bone mass. Medications such as steroids may also have a detrimental effect on the achievement of peak bone mass.

BONE LOSS

Bone density usually plateaus from age thirty to the late forties, especially in the spine, but there might be some hip loss even at this stage in life. This may be related to a reduction in physical activity levels. A much more dramatic reduction in bone mass occurs at around the time of menopause or a few years earlier, perhaps related to declining estrogen levels. Men do not have this rapid bone loss because they do not experience any such dramatic, complete decline in either estrogen (female hormone) or testosterone (male hormone) levels. This helps protect men from osteoporosis (in addition to the fact that peak bone mass levels relative to bone area are higher in men than women). However, with advancing age (seventy years and above), levels in both hormones may decline somewhat and cause some of the age-related bone loss in men.

Approximately after the age of thirty, some bone loss occurs in everyone, although the rates of loss vary. Some might ask: If bone loss occurs in everybody, why don't all of us get osteoporosis? Well, if we all lived long enough and didn't treat ourselves with bone-protective medicines, we probably all would get osteoporosis. Second, osteoporosis-related fractures are extremely common; almost one in two white women, for instance, will have a fracture from osteoporosis at some point in her lifetime. The likelihood of getting osteoporosis depends on the amount of bone achieved at peak and the rate and duration of bone loss. Most people who have low peak bone mass and a high rate of bone loss are going to develop osteoporosis. Those who have a high peak bone mass and slow rate of loss are the least likely to get osteoporosis; only a small percentage will. All others have an intermediate risk. Again, since we cannot actually determine amount of bone loss unless a bone mass measurement is made at the time that peak skeletal mass is attained (young adulthood), all these factors are theoretical and have to be inferred based on the medical and family history that a person can provide.

WHY DOES BONE LOSS OCCUR?

Bone is actually a living tissue. Many mistakenly think bones are like fingernails. But this is wrong. Unlike fingernails, which don't have cells, blood vessels, or nerves, bones have all three. In fact, there are three different types of cells in bones. Bones encase bone marrow, a highly active organ of the body responsible for making blood cells. Bone undergoes a constant rejuvenation process called bone remodeling, which involves cells located in the bone marrow. Bone as an organ is thus completely distinct from nails or hair, which do not have cells and do not undergo remodeling. New nails and hair emanate from living nail beds and hair follicles, but nails and hair themselves are not alive. This is why cutting nails and hair produces no pain.

It is thought that the bone remodeling process protects the skeleton from the effects of accumulated fatigue damage. In other words, remodeling occurs after bone becomes old or weak or accumulates minor cracks or microscopic damage, which can ultimately undermine its strength. That piece of bone that has this minor damage becomes dissolved or resorbed by cells called osteoclasts, which are recruited to the area by certain attractant chemicals from cells called osteocytes that sense when a bone is damaged. After the osteoclasts have removed the damaged piece of bone, they disappear, and bone-forming cells made from precursor cells in the bone marrow are recruited to the area, probably also by chemical attractants. The osteoblasts form a new section of bone to replace what was removed by the osteoclasts (see figure 3-2).

During youth and young adulthood, the amount of bone that is resorbed is balanced by the same amount of bone being formed. This balance is upset during later adulthood, particularly at the time of menopause and with advancing age. In menopausal women, the bone resorption part of remodeling becomes particularly aggressive: The cells that break down bone—the osteoclasts—rapidly dig out deep cavities from bone. The cells that make bone, the osteoblasts, cannot keep up, and at every microscopic remodeling unit there occurs a small amount of bone loss. Furthermore, while digging these deep holes, the osteoclasts can actually perforate some of the cross-connecting pieces of bone, called the trabeculae. As a re-

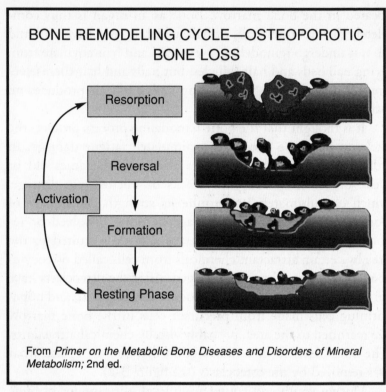

BONE REMODELING CYCLE—OSTEOPOROTIC BONE LOSS

From *Primer on the Metabolic Bone Diseases and Disorders of Mineral Metabolism;* 2nd ed.

Figure 3-2: Throughout life, bone undergoes a constant rejuvenation process called bone remodeling. In menopausal women, the cells that break down bone rapidly dig out deep cavities, while the cells that make bone cannot keep up.

sult of these perforations, the whole microarchitecture of bone becomes disordered. If you imagine a three-dimensional lattice structure with holes in it or a particularly porous piece of Swiss cheese, this is what happens to bone after the aggressive remodeling at the time of menopause. (See figures 3-3 A and B.) In fact, osteoporosis is defined not only by reduced mass of bone tissue, but also by a disruption in the microscopic structure of bone. Also at menopause, the amount of the skeleton undergoing remodeling at any time is dramatically increased. Bone loss is caused, therefore, by the small amount of bone lost at each remodeling unit and the existence of many more remodeling units at any one time. Strategies to combat osteoporosis, therefore, include returning bone remodeling levels to normal, preventing bone loss, and in some cases improving the efficiency or magnitude of osteoblast activity, thereby increasing bone formation.

As noted, the balance within the bone remodeling cycle becomes upset with age. The osteoblasts (bone-forming cells) cannot replace bone as efficiently and/or suffer an earlier demise. As a result, the amount of bone removed during remodeling

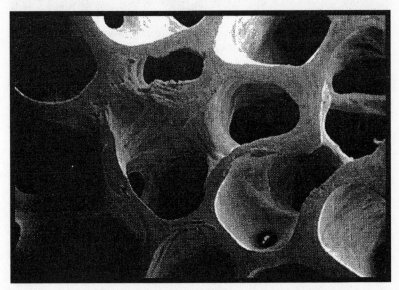

Figure 3-3A: Normal cancellous or "spongy" bone. Reprinted from *J Bone Miner Res* 1986; 1:15–21 with permission of the American Society for Bone and Mineral Research.

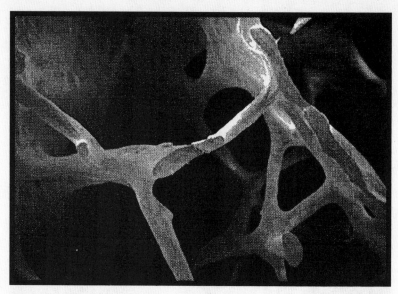

Figure 3-3B: Osteoporotic bone. Reprinted from *J Bone Miner Res* 1986; 1:15-21 with permission of the American Society for Bone and Mineral Research.

cannot be completely replaced. Thus an ongoing age-related bone loss occurs in both men and women after the accelerated bone loss of the first five years after menopause. It's possible to actually measure the activity of the bone-forming cells by looking at bone biopsy specimens under the microscope.

While bone loss is inevitable with menopause and age, the rate of loss differs among individuals, and is influenced by a number of environmental as well as genetic factors. A low life-long calcium intake and poor exercise habits, as well as smoking and excessive alcohol ingestion, increase the rate of loss. Certain medications can also increase rates of bone loss and fracture occurrence, including the steroids or glucocorticoids used to treat autoimmune or inflammatory diseases, particularly rheumatoid arthritis (but not osteoarthritis, the most common wear-and-tear-type joint disease), lupus, inflammatory bowel disease (but not irritable bowel), and asthma or other chronic obstructive lung disease. Some of these diseases increase the rate of bone loss even if steroids are not used, particularly rheumatoid arthritis and inflammatory bowel disease (ulcerative colitis, or Crohn's disease). Many other diseases, including malabsorption disorders such as celiac disease (gluten-sensitive enteropathy); neurologic diseases including stroke, Parkinson's disease, and multiple sclerosis; certain endocrine or hormonal disorders (some types of diabetes, as well as overactive thyroid or parathyroid glands); and various genetic diseases, all increase bone loss.

BONE QUALITY

Some factors that can influence the strength of bone and ability to resist fracturing cannot be measured easily. As mentioned earlier, when the osteoclasts dig aggressively at bone tissue at menopause, there may be perforation of some of the cross-connecting pieces of bone, called trabeculae. Imagine a piece of Jarlsberg cheese where holes have actually bored completely through some of the indentations. These perforations can have a big influence on bone strength even if the mass of tissue is only minimally affected. Furthermore, the presence of ditches on the bone surface may be a point of weakness and lead to increased risk of fracturing. The age of bone is also thought to have an influence on strength. For example, in various rare bone diseases (such as one called osteopetrosis), in which the remodeling process is impaired and old, slightly damaged bone cannot be repaired, fractures are common, even though the amount of bone tissue is normal.

FALLING RISK

A high frequency of falls is a determinant of fracture risk. Most falls do not produce fractures, even when bone density is low, but obviously, in a person who does have osteoporosis, the more falls that occur, the more likely it is that one of them is going to be serious enough to cause a fracture. Any neurologic or muscle diseases that produce weakness or problems with balance can increase the risk of falling. Diseases that produce seizures or fainting spells similarly increase the risk of fracture. Medications used to treat anxiety, depression, or pain; induce sleep; and treat high blood pressure and diabetes may also result in an increased risk of falls.

The young man with very severe osteoporosis whom I described earlier was using a large amount of medication to treat his severe chronic back pain. Although he was using a walker to help him get from room to room, he became drowsy as a result of the narcotic medication and fell asleep while trying to get to the bathroom. The resulting fall was the cause of the hip fracture that soon afterward took his life. Perhaps if he had used less sedating medicine or had assistance while going to the bathroom, the fall would have been prevented and he would have lived. Certainly, estimating and reducing the risk of osteoporosis entails reviewing the need for any medication, making sure that the dose used is the lowest possible, and determining whether there could be interactions among medications that could result in excessive drowsiness, sedation, dizziness, or the like.

Another factor increasing falls is a lack of good environmental safety precautions: poor lighting, particularly in the hallway to the bathroom, wires or strings from curtains lying on the floor, movable furniture, throw rugs without friction surfaces on the bottom, wearing socks on slippery tile or wood floors, and spills on tile or wood floors. Excessively long clothing can produce trips, particularly when going up stairs. Shoes with slippery soles cause falls. Every day I see patients who have had serious fractures resulting from falls that could have been avoided by taking a little more care to ensure a safe environment. Move slowly and take pride in creating the safest possible environment to reduce the risk of injury!

THE BARE BONES

- Bone mass accumulates during youth, even after height maxes out, and peaks between ages twenty and thirty.
- Peak bone mass is largely a function of genetic makeup, but nutrition, exercise, integrity of menstrual function, and a healthy lifestyle also play a role.
- Bone is a living tissue that is constantly undergoing a renewal process. When the rate of bone dissolution exceeds the amount of bone formation, bone loss occurs.
- Though bone loss at menopause and with advancing age is inevitable, rates of loss can be slowed by preventive measures.
- Fracture risk in adults is related to bone density; bone density in later adulthood is a function of the amount of bone attained in young adulthood minus the amount of bone subsequently lost.
- Fracture risk also depends on bone quality and frequency of falling.

Part II

PREVENTING
AND
SLOWING
THE EFFECTS
OF OSTEOPOROSIS

Chapter 4

Prevention:
The Universal Message

The skeleton has a number of very important functions. It gives our bodies their major shape, keeping us upright on our feet and allowing us to walk and to move all our extremities. It also surrounds and protects our inner organs. The skull protects the brain, and the spine protects the spinal cord. The ribs protect the heart, lungs, and upper abdominal organs such as the liver and spleen. The skeleton also provides a milieu for the bone marrow, or tissue, that produces white blood cells, red blood cells, and platelets. It is therefore critical to keep our bones healthy; not only will this prevent fractures, but by preventing fractures it will ultimately also allow the skeleton to perform all of its intended functions.

The earlier we begin taking care of our bones, the more likely we are to benefit. Bone health begins in infancy and young childhood. This is similar to precepts regarding the prevention of other chronic diseases. When it comes to heart disease prevention, for instance, the earlier we begin a low-saturated-fat diet and regular exercise, the more impact it will ultimately have on preventing the accumulation of fatty atherosclerotic deposits in our arteries. And the earlier in life we begin consuming lots of cancer-fighting vegetables and fruits, the more likely we will have an impact on prevention of cancer.

This is not to imply, however, that lifestyle choices can overwhelm the importance of genetics. As mentioned in chapter 3, the major determinant of osteoporosis risk is our genetic makeup. We cannot assume that osteoporosis can be completely prevented. It is important for people to realize that even if they have been doing everything possible to improve their skeletal health, they might develop osteoporosis. The upper limit of peak bone mass for each individual (usually attained by the age of twenty-five years) is probably determined by genetic factors. If the appropriate health promotion or prevention measures are followed, individuals should be able to reach their genetic potential—but this might still be lower than normal due to predominant genetic factors. Women and men at risk (based on their family history, low body weight, low dietary calcium intake, sedentary lifestyle, smoking, or heavy drinking) must get bone density tests (see chapter 10)—the only means by which osteoporosis can be diagnosed in its early stages—prior to the development of fractures. By stressing lifestyle choices, we are empowering ourselves to at least do everything we can to keep our bones as healthy as we can. Once we accomplish this, if something goes wrong, we cannot be blamed. It is important to accept that some things are out of our hands; we are not responsible for every illness that hits us. We cannot blame the victim.

The following three chapters provide the information we need to do everything possible to prevent osteoporosis. It is never too late to begin caring for our bones. The importance of healthy lifestyle, nutrition, and exercise can be demonstrated even very late in life, in terms of both bone mass and fractures.

THE BARE BONES

- The consequences of osteoporosis generally do not occur until later in life, but damage to the skeleton usually begins many years earlier.
- All women and men—as well as adolescents and young children—should learn what they can do to prevent chronic diseases, including osteoporosis.
- The earlier that prevention measures are taken, the more impact they will have on reducing future risk of disease. Still, it's never too late to develop bone-healthy behaviors.
- The cornerstones of prevention are reducing risk factors, optimizing nutrition, and exercising regularly.
- If you have a genetic predisposition to osteoporosis, even if you practice all the osteoporosis prevention measures throughout your life, you may still develop the condition.

Chapter 5

Prevention Step One:
Reducing Risk Factors

One of the most important factors in preventing osteoporosis is eliminating or reducing risk factors. This chapter describes the measures—including lifestyle choices, safety practices, and medications—that can be modified to reduce the risk of osteoporosis.

SMOKING

First and foremost on the list of habits offensive to the skeleton is smoking. Smoking increases the risk of hip fracture by 100 percent. For example, if the lifetime risk of hip fracture on average is 15 percent, a smoker has an average lifetime risk of 30 percent. Smoking has direct toxic effects on the cells that make bone. It also reduces estrogen levels and can result in an earlier menopause. Smokers are overall less physically active, and a sedentary lifestyle is another risk for the development of osteoporosis. Furthermore, there is evidence that quitting smoking is an important way to reduce fracture risk. Women who stop smoking can cut their hip fracture risk in half after five years. This is similar to the impact of smoking on heart disease: Again, cessation can reduce the risk substantially within five years. Preventing osteoporosis is just another of the myriad reasons why people should quit smoking.

MEDICATIONS

A large group of medicines can influence bone health, reduce acquisition of peak bone mass, or increase the amount of bone loss. These include, most importantly, steroids and thyroid hormone. Sometimes these medicines are started with questionable indications. In some cases, it may not be possible to eliminate these medications; still, any reduction in the dose might help benefit bone.

Steroids (also called glucocorticoids or corticosteroids) are medications such as prednisone, cortisone, and medrol. They are usually taken by mouth as pills but also come in forms for intravenous use and in inhalers for use in patients with asthma and other chronic lung diseases. Besides lung diseases, these sometimes lifesaving medications are used for a variety of autoimmune diseases—those in which the body attacks itself because it mistakenly perceives itself as something foreign. Some of the most common conditions for which they are used besides asthma and emphysema (chronic obstructive lung disease) are rheumatoid arthritis, lupus, polymyalgia rheumatica, multiple sclerosis, inflammatory bowel disease (ulcerative colitis, Crohn's disease), and certain cancers. Unfortunately, there are often no alternative treatments for some of these illnesses. Where there are alternatives that can be tried safely, they should be. The doses of steroid should be the lowest possible to control the illness, and they should be stopped as soon as your doctor believes possible. The inhalers should be used instead of pills, when possible, since these have less of a detrimental effect on bone and other organ systems.

With thyroid hormone, there is one rare indication for use in which large doses are required: among people who have had thyroid cancer. Here the hormone is used to shut down the releasing hormone from the pituitary gland. Normally, the pituitary gland produces a small amount of the hormone to stimulate the thyroid gland. In people who have had thyroid cancer, however, it may be important to prevent any stimulation of the remaining thyroid tissue. Some patients are treated with thyroid hormone to try to suppress the growth of small benign tumors called nodules. This makes sense in some individuals, but many times the thyroid medication is started and the nodule is never reassessed. It would not be reasonable to remain on a high dose of thyroid hormone forever to prevent growth of a benign nodule. It is important to discuss the pros and cons with your doctor every six months.

Most people are actually started on thyroid medicine to replace what their own glands are not making, a condition called hypothyroidism. This may occur as a result of prior surgery or treatment of the overactive condition (Graves' disease) or be due to an autoimmune disease called Hashimoto's disease. Endocrinologists who specialize in treatment of this condition usually perform a blood test called the TSH level every three to six months to determine very carefully the dose of thyroid hormone needed to replace what the patient's thyroid is not making. This is very important for two reasons: The dose needed can vary, and overdose can cause serious complications for the skeleton and elsewhere. In bone, excessive amounts of thyroid hormone can accelerate bone loss and increase the risk of fractures. In contrast, correct amounts of thyroid hormone will not produce any adverse effects on bone. In short, anyone on thyroid hormone should be sure to get a blood test periodically to make sure that the dose of the medicine is appropriate.

Antiseizure medications, immunosuppressive drugs such as methotrexate, and chemotherapy agents for various cancers can all adversely affect bone. Obviously, in these cases, the importance of controlling the primary disease with any means possible almost always exceeds the importance of any adverse effect on bone. It is important to realize that a bone density test should be done as early as possible after menopause in women who have used these medicines for a significant period of time—say, six months or more. This will allow treatment for osteoporosis to be started early in people at high risk.

ALCOHOL

Excessive alcohol intake is associated with a dramatic impact on bone mass. Alcoholics have terrible osteoporosis. The reasons are probably multiple and include poor overall nutrition, including suboptimal calcium intake. Alcoholics also tend to have poor exercise habits. Alcohol might directly affect bone cells and impair their ability to re-form bone during the normal remodeling cycle. Alcoholics who already have osteoporosis are at further risk of fracturing because they often fall or experience other minor or major accidents. The prevention and treatment of osteoporosis must always include treatment of alcohol abuse if it is present.

Modest or moderate amounts of alcohol ingestion, however, do not have a negative effect on bone. In fact, small amounts of alcohol might actually increase bone mass—perhaps by increasing average estrogen levels, though there may be other reasons as well. With bone, alcohol consumption has effects similar to what we see with the heart. Low to moderate doses seems to be healthful, but large and excessive doses are clearly harmful. Of course, we don't want to advocate alcohol ingestion for everyone, especially since it might be difficult to know who is at risk for alcoholism. Those who drink a little with no excessive consumption should not change.

HOW TO REDUCE YOUR CHANCE OF FALLING

Since most fractures occur in the context of a fall, specifically introducing efforts to reduce the likelihood of falling could make a substantial impact on osteoporosis prevention. The likelihood of falls increases dramatically by the midsixties, and people with a history of falling are much more likely to fall again. Any patients who have had recent multiple falls or who feel light-headed, dizzy, or unsteady on their feet should have a medical evaluation to search for a cause. This should begin with an internist and may involve cardiac and neurologic consultations and evaluations. A referral to a physical therapist who can evaluate gait might be beneficial for a specific balance-and-coordination program or for consideration of an ambulation assistive device such as a cane or walker. Many older people are self-conscious about these devices; however, they can be enormously beneficial to quality of life and overall health if they keep people mobile, while avoiding falls.

Reducing the risk of falls—particularly in elderly women and men—includes reviewing medicines that cause sleepiness or sedation, dizziness, or drop in blood pressure. Among these are medicines affecting the central nervous system (antidepressants, anti-anxiety medicines, medicines to induce sleep), blood pressure medicines, water pills, and medicines to control blood sugar. Stopping or reducing the dose of any such medicine, when this is possible, could help reduce risk of falling. Therefore, one of the first steps toward reducing falling risk is to review your medicines with your doctor. Ask:

- Are all of your medications necessary?
- Are they being used in the lowest possible doses?
- Are there any drug combinations that might make you particularly prone to light-headedness?

Vision and hearing problems can contribute to falling risk. Problems with depth perception might be particularly culpable. Anything that can be done to improve these factors should be done:

- A person whose vision is significantly impaired by cataracts should get them removed.
- Lens prescriptions should be checked for adequacy by an optometrist or ophthalmologist.
- Patients with diabetes or high blood pressure, who are especially prone to abnormalities of the retina and the resulting visual deterioration, should have an eye examination by an ophthalmologist to determine if any improvements can be achieved with retinal procedures.
- Hearing loss should be evaluated by an audiologist, and hearing aids should be used and adjusted as needed.

It is also very important, particularly for older people, to review the safety of the home environment:

- Hallways should be well lit, especially those used at night on the way to the bathroom.
- Lights should be within easy reach of the bed.

- There should be no cords or wires dangling in footpaths that could precipitate tripping.
- Do not rest or stabilize yourself on mobile furniture such as small tables on wheels.
- Avoid throw rugs unless they have a very good friction surface at the bottom.
- Walking-assistive devices such as canes or walkers should be readily accessible when you get out of bed to reduce the risk of falling on the way to the bathroom.
- Place rubber or adhesive strips in the bathtub or shower.
- Assess clothing for safety; shoes should have nonslip surfaces, and hemlines should be short enough to prevent tripping.
- Handrails should be available on all stairways.
- Cracks or uneven sidewalk surfaces should be repaired.
- Driveways should be well lit.
- Use common sense regarding inclement weather. Obviously, freezing rain or icy surfaces are the cause of many winter falls, and outdoor activities are hazardous in these conditions.

NORMAL MENSTRUAL FUNCTION

In young women, abnormal menstrual function may be associated with lower bone mass. Very infrequent menstrual periods or long intervals without menses may be a sign of inadequate estrogen levels in the body. This in turn can be related to genetic factors; certain diseases, including the eating disorder anorexia nervosa; or very excessive exercise, such as might be present among long-distance runners, gymnasts, or semiprofessional or professional ballet dancers. All these conditions may be associated with reduced bone mass and a greater likelihood of osteoporosis. Usually, prevention of bone loss in these conditions begins with treatment of the underlying disease. The sooner anorexia nervosa is suspected, the more likely it can be treated effectively. This must involve adequate nutrition, weight gain, major psychological counseling, and sometimes medication. While the use of oral contraceptive medication has been advocated by some for prevention of bone loss in anorexia, oral contraceptives alone will not do much to help the skeletal or other complications of this horrific illness. Young women who are not menstruating most months due to genetic factors (such as Turner's syndrome) might benefit from oral contraceptive medications for estrogen repletion. It is not clear whether using oral contraceptives will benefit bone mass in adolescents or young women who are overtraining for semi-professional or professional athletic endeavors. Reducing training and perhaps allowing a bit of increased weight can help, but these measures are often resisted because they might negatively impact performance in this elite category.

THE BARE BONES

- Your risk factors for bone loss and falling must be addressed as the first step toward osteoporosis prevention.
- If you smoke, quit! Use whatever is necessary: medications, therapy, hypnosis, acupuncture, or support groups.
- Alcohol abuse must be identified and treated.
- If you take thyroid hormone, you must be evaluated with regular blood tests (TSH levels) to ensure that the dose is not excessive. If the reasons for initiating the thyroid hormone were dubious to begin with (based on symptoms without confirmatory blood tests), speak to your doctor

about tapering and discontinuing medication if symptoms and blood tests permit.

- If you take steroids, you should discuss options with your doctor and make sure that you are on the lowest possible doses to control your illness. If you are on steroids for asthma or related conditions, you may be able to try steroid inhalers, which are less detrimental to bone health.

- Decrease your falling risk by evaluating medications, vision or hearing impairment, and nervous system or heart disease.

- Evaluate your home for safety hazards and make the modifications necessary to reduce falling risk.

- If you are a young woman who has very infrequent menstrual periods, you should talk to your doctor.

Chapter 6

Prevention Step Two: Nutrition

Proper nutrition is incredibly important to bone health and osteoporosis prevention. During childhood and adolescence, this includes adequate calories and protein as well as calcium and vitamin D. These nutrients are the building blocks of the skeleton. Since the skeleton is involved in constant renewal, and some nutrients are excreted by the body, we need to continue to supply them on a daily basis.

This chapter will review current concepts about optimal nutrition for bone health, concentrating on adequate calcium and vitamin D intake, with the use of supplements if necessary. The evidence for effects of other supplements (besides calcium and vitamin D) on bone health will be discussed in chapter 8.

CALCIUM

Adequate calcium intake can help protect bones throughout life. In childhood and during the teen years, an adequate calcium intake can help produce a higher peak bone mass. Peak bone mass is the peak amount of bone an individual ever attains, usually by the age of twenty-five. In young adulthood (through the early forties), an adequate calcium intake can help maintain bone density, especially in the hip, where some loss can occur. Among perimenopausal, postmenopausal, and aged women, adequate calcium intake reduces rates of bone loss though it may not completely prevent bone loss.

It is normal to lose some calcium daily in our excretions (both urine and feces) as well as in our sweat and through our lungs when we breathe. Therefore we need to consume enough calcium each day to make up for these losses. For most healthy individuals, following the calcium recommendations below should make up for these daily losses. If the calcium requirements are not met, the body will take calcium from the bones, which serve as the major storage pool for calcium, to maintain adequate levels in the blood. Maintaining these levels is critical for the normal functioning of the heart and arteries, nerves, and muscles. The body will sacrifice the skeleton (allow it to become weak and susceptible to fractures), if it needs to, in order to maintain these other more immediately life-threatening bodily functions.

RECOMMENDED CALCIUM INTAKES

Recommended calcium intakes vary throughout your life (see figure 6-1). Calcium intake is likely to be adequate in infancy from both breast milk and formulas as long as calorie consumption is adequate and babies are growing as expected. During the toddler years, an intake of slightly less than two eight-ounce glasses of milk each day or equivalent servings of cheese, yogurt, or calcium-fortified foods should suffice. In early-childhood years (ages four through eight), a bit more calcium is required:

Optimal Calcium Intakes

Age in Years	Daily Calcium Needed
1–3	500 mg
4–8	800 mg
9–18	1,300 mg
19–50	1,000 mg
51 or older	1,200 mg

Dietary Reference Intakes, National Academy of Science, 1997.

Figure 6-1.

at least two servings a day of calcium-dense foods. Adequate calcium throughout late childhood (ages nine through eighteen) should be the highest at any phase in life (1,300 mg), because this is the time when adolescents are growing rapidly in terms of both bone length or height and also consolidating bone mineral. This latter effect means that the amount of bone and bone mineral is actually increasing within a fixed volume. In fact, it is during this time that fractures, such as those of the wrist, can occur commonly. One explanation of this phenomenon is that children who are not getting adequate dietary calcium to support normal growth might be taking some from the distal wrist to supply enough for linear growth especially during growth spurts. Once the growth spurts are complete, the bone is put back into the wrist and the likelihood of fracturing becomes less. During young adulthood (ages nineteen through fifty), a total calcium intake of 1,000 mg per day is enough. Thereafter, from age fifty-one, the calcium requirements remain stable for the rest of life at about 1,200 mg per day. Three or more servings of calcium-dense foods (dairy and/or highly fortified foods), plus the calcium from trace sources (vegetables, grains, nuts, and others), is usually enough to obtain the recommended daily calcium.

DIETARY INFLUENCES OF OTHER NUTRIENTS ON CALCIUM BALANCE

The calcium contained in food we eat is digested in the stomach, then moved into the small intestine where it is absorbed into the blood for use by the body. Certain foods can decrease the absorption of calcium. These include caffeine, wheat fiber, phytates, oxalates, and supplemental iron. Excessive caffeine should perhaps be avoided for other reasons, though moderate caffeine consumption is probably not detrimental to health. In contrast, wheat fiber is an important part of the diet as it might help maintain lower cholesterol levels and might also be good for colon health maintenance. If you add supplemental fiber, try to get your calcium-dense foods at a different time. Foods containing phytates include beans, peas, seeds, nuts, and cereal grains. Oxalates are found in spinach, sweet potato, rhubarb, swiss chard, and beans. There is no reason from the perspective of the skeleton to avoid consumption of these products, however, since they have important nutrient value and an otherwise adequate calcium intake will be able to overcome any small influence of these nutrients on calcium absorption. For example, the calcium from spinach is not well absorbed; however, any other calcium eaten with the spinach will be well absorbed. Iron pills or vitamins containing iron should not be taken with calcium since calcium and iron interfere with each other's absorption.

Other influences on calcium balance in the body include salt and protein. Excessive consumption of these products might increase the amount of calcium excreted in the urine. Again, however, current calcium recommendations should be able to compensate for average American consumption of both. In general, many Americans are eating too much salt and meat protein anyway, so reducing intake might be warranted for purposes completely separate from bone health, such as heart and blood vessel health. Much ado has been made of the issue of phosphates in soda, particularly colas, and their influence on calcium absorption and bone. In fact, the influence of phosphates on calcium balance is minimal or nil; the problem is rather that many adolescents and adults who drink lots of soda also drink very little milk and eat very few dairy products and other calcium-dense foods. If calcium intake is adequate, then there will be no adverse effect of soda or cola consumption on bone health.

OBTAINING CALCIUM FROM FOOD

It is often possible, if wise food choices are made, to obtain the optimal calcium intake from food. Dairy products contain the highest density of calcium per serving. These include milk, yogurt, and cheese as well as cheese-containing mixed dishes. The soy-based and rice-based milks, yogurts, tofu, and cheeses are available fortified to contain amounts of calcium similar to those of cow-based dairy products. Canned fish products with bones (salmon, sardines) also contain a generous amount of calcium; fresh fish fillets without bones, however, are not a significant source. Some vegetables contain significant amounts of calcium, particularly bok choy; dandelion, turnip, and mustard greens; kale; artichokes; and broccoli. Many other foods contain small amounts of calcium, including baked beans, oranges, figs, almonds, and hummus. A list of the calcium contents of certain foods is provided in figure 6-2.

Calcium Content of Dairy Foods and
High-Calcium Nondairy Alternatives

Dairy Foods

Food	Serving	Calcium
Carnation Instant Breakfast	1 packet	500 mg
Yogurt	1 cup	200–400 mg
Ricotta cheese	¼ cup	250–300 mg
Milk	8 ounces	300 mg
Mixed-cheese dishes (1 serving = 1 slice pizza, 1 cup macaroni and cheese, or 1 cup lasagna)	1 serving	200 mg
Cheese, sliced or shredded	1 ounce	175–270 mg
Creamed soup, made with milk	1 cup	165–190 mg
Cheese, string	1 ounce	150–200 mg
Cream cheese	2 tablespoons	150 mg
Pudding	½ cup	150 mg
Frozen yogurt	½ cup	100–200 mg
Ice cream	½ cup	80–150 mg
Ice pop (fudge, yogurt)	1	100 mg
Cottage cheese	½ cup	60–100 mg
Parmesan cheese	1 tablespoon	40–60 mg

Bread, Cereal, Rice, and Pasta Group

Pancakes	⅛ cup batter	100–200 mg
Tortilla, flour or corn	1 6-inch	45 mg

Fats, Oils, and Sweets (Use Sparingly)

Molasses, blackstrap	1 tablespoon	170 mg

Meats, Poultry, Fish, Dry Beans, Eggs, and Nuts Group

Food	Serving	Calcium
Sardines, canned with bones	4 ounces	350 mg
Salmon, canned with bones	3 ounces	200 mg
Cheeseburger	3 ounces	100–150 mg
Egg substitute	½ cup	130 mg
Canned beans	½ cup	40–60 mg
Almonds	1 ounce	80 mg
Hummus	½ cup	60 mg
Egg	1	30 mg

Vegetable Group

Food	Serving	Calcium
Turnip greens, cooked	1 cup	200 mg
Bok choy, cooked	1 cup	160 mg
Dandelion greens, cooked	1 cup	140 mg
Artichoke, boiled	1 medium	135 mg
Mustard greens, cooked	1 cup	105 mg
Kale, cooked	1 cup	100 mg
Broccoli, cooked	1 cup	70 mg
Broccoli, raw	1 cup	40 mg

Figure 6-2.

There are some zealots who believe that milk is the only way, and other zealots who believe that milk is terribly detrimental to health. Neither is correct, and both are irresponsible in their vociferous campaigns in lay publications and advertisements. As specified above and below, there are many ways to get calcium besides milk. I would agree with the latter group that whole milk is not particularly healthy, given its high saturated-fat content. But 1 percent fat milk or completely fat-free milk are excellent choices for calcium. Regarding those who are on the ban-milk campaign, they often claim in their argument that milk exerts detrimental effects on bone. They have misinterpreted the data concerning the protein content in milk. They believe that the protein in milk will "leach out" the calcium. As I mentioned above, while animal and vegetable proteins might result in a slight increase in urine calcium, they are not bad for the skeleton. In fact, inadequate protein intake, especially in the elderly, has been shown to be a risk factor for hip fracture, and protein supplementation can improve recovery after hip fracture surgery. And certainly milk, because of its high calcium content, is beneficial for bone. The calcium in milk is highly bioavailable (absorbable and usable by the body). Some critics draw upon studies showing that people who have a high milk or calcium consumption have a higher risk of hip fracture. These studies are primarily retrospective, meaning that the subjects were questioned about their milk and calcium intake after having had a hip fracture. This is a case of trying to figure out which came first, the chicken or the egg. In many cases, people increase their milk and calcium consumption *after* having fractures. It might therefore look as if high calcium consumption is associated with increased fracture occurrence. In contrast, perhaps if these individuals had increased their calcium consumption for a substantial time prior to the fracture, the fracture might not have occurred.

CALCIUM-FORTIFIED FOODS

One of the greatest advances in osteoporosis prevention and treatment is the proliferation of calcium-fortified foods (foods with calcium added), which are now available on almost all shelves of the supermarket. This has made it much easier to obtain the appropriate intake from dietary sources. There are some individuals who simply do not like milk or milk products. My oldest daughter is one of these. She cannot drink milk as a beverage (it makes her gag) or eat yogurt. Nor does she like cheese or macaroni with cheese, a staple for many children. (I don't think this is my fault, because I have two other children who love chocolate milk, yogurt, and cheese.) Instead, she eats lots of calcium-fortified cereal (with plenty of fat-free milk), calcium-fortified juices, calcium-fortified hot cocoa (from dry mix), and calcium-fortified waffles and other breakfast and snack bars.

A lot of people are confused about how to select calcium-fortified foods, because calcium content varies substantially among different products. See figure 6-3 for a partial listing of fortified foods with their calcium contents. For example, calcium-fortified citrus juices have between 300 and 400 mg of calcium per serving—as much or more than the same quantity of milk. This is also true with certain waffles. Some calcium-fortified cereals have even more calcium per serving than milk—up to 1,000 mg per serving—while some have only 100 mg per serving. Similarly, some kids' juices and juice boxes, as well as many snack foods (crackers and graham crackers), contain about 100 mg per serving. Hot cocoa mixes can have between 100 and 300 mg per serving, and Carnation Instant Breakfast provides a walloping 500. Certain cheese and cracker snack packs have up to 300 mg. Even at the lower level of calcium fortification, 100 mg per serving, these foods can go a long way toward helping kids (and adults) obtain the correct amount of calcium. Due to the variability in calcium content, it is essential to look carefully at the nutrition information for each product and to add up the calcium content accordingly. See figure 6-4 for help in reading calcium content from food labels.

Fortified Foods at a Glance*

Food	Serving	Calcium
Milk	8 ounces	400 mg
Cottage cheese	½ cup	120–200 mg
Vegetable juice	8 ounces	300 mg
Cereal	1 serving	100–1,000 mg
Hot cereal	1 packet	100–350 mg
Waffles	2	100–300 mg
Cheese crackers	1 serving	100–250 mg
Cheese and cracker snacks	1 package	300 mg
Graham crackers	2	100 mg
Bread	1 slice	50 mg
Juice drinks	8 ounces	100 mg
Citrus juices	8 ounces	300–350 mg
Cereal/snack bars	1 bar	200–250 mg
Milk chocolate granola bars	1 serving	200 mg
Cookies	1 serving	100 mg

Soy Products (Calcium-Fortified)

Soy yogurt	6 ounces	500 mg
Soy or rice milk	8 ounces	200–300 mg
Soy cheese	1 slice	200 mg
Tofu	⅛ block	300 mg
Soy nuts	½ cup	230 mg
Soy cakes	1 serving	100–250 mg

*All of these products are not naturally high in calcium but can be purchased in calcium-fortified or -enriched forms. You must check the label to ensure that you are getting the fortified product.

Figure 6-3.

Reading Food Labels for Calcium Content

The calcium content of foods varies widely depending upon growing conditions (fruits, vegetables, and legumes), brand, and amount of calcium added to fortified foods. Reading the food label is an easy way to find out how much calcium is in one serving of food. It can help you select foods that contain the most calcium.

Food labels do not list calcium in milligrams. Instead, the label lists % Daily Value (% DV) for calcium in each serving. One hundred percent of the DV for calcium is equal to 1000 mg of calcium per day.

To find the calcium content (mg per serving) from % Daily Value:

1. Read the % DV for calcium per serving. For example: 1 serving (1 ounce) lowfat cheese contains 20% calcium.

2. Simply drop the "%" from the DV and add a "0" to the end of the Daily Value number (or multiply by 10). For example, 20% calcium = 200 mg calcium.

Figure 6-4.

HOW DOES ADEQUATE DIETARY CALCIUM FIT IN WITH OTHER DIETARY RECOMMENDATIONS?

Adequate dietary calcium does not interfere with other important healthful diet measures. Everyone agrees that we should be eating more fruits (two to four daily servings) and vegetables (three to five daily servings). In fact, these can be good calcium sources if you choose calcium-fortified vegetable, tomato, or citrus juices, or if you eat high-calcium-content green vegetables such as bok choy, broccoli, and kale. Fruit is a great snack, but there is some evidence that carbohydrates by themselves might produce rapid increases in blood sugar levels that are not ultimately healthy. Adding a piece of reduced-fat cheese, some low-fat yogurt or milk, or a serving of high-calcium-content nuts, such as almonds or roasted soy nuts, can help prevent such rapid increases in blood sugar and also provide some calcium. The same is true of the grain products that are currently at the bottom of the food pyramid. It may not be so healthy to eat these products plain, in the absence of protein. Add low-fat cheese, milk, or yogurt, and they become much healthier. Sprinkle Parmesan cheese on pasta, instead of butter; you're adding more protein and calcium and reducing the fat a bit. In any event, it's definitely possible to get enough calcium and maintain a good basic diet.

ESTIMATING DIETARY CALCIUM

To make sure you are getting enough calcium in your diet (and to determine how to modify it, or whether a supplement is necessary), a quick estimate of dietary calcium content can be made. Figure 6-5 shows an easy way to calculate your calcium intake. Calcium-containing dairy foods should be low fat or nonfat to meet standards for optimal cardiovascular health. Dairy foods contain an average of 300 mg per serving. Calcium-fortified foods comprise the next largest amount of calcium in the diet.

Other sources of calcium in the diet, such as green vegetables, nuts, grain products, and certain fruits, contain smaller quantities of calcium or tend to be consumed too infrequently to be included in a quick, easy estimate of daily calcium intake. The average American diet contains about 250 mg per day from these nondairy, nonfortified sources. If you are an individual who consumes large amounts of some of these products, you can add in the amounts of calcium (see figure 6-2) from the frequently eaten foods to determine your average calcium intake. You must then omit the 250 mg addition for trace dietary calcium sources.

Estimating Daily Dietary Calcium Intake

Product	# of Servings		Calcium Content	Calcium (mg)
Milk (8 oz.)	_____	x	300 mg/serving =	_____
Yogurt (8 oz.)	_____	x	400 mg/serving =	_____
Cheese (1 oz.)	_____	x	200 mg/serving =	_____
Fortified citrus* juice (8 oz.)	_____	x	300 mg/serving =	_____
Fortified cereal* and other fortified foods*	_____	x	100–1,000 mg/serving =	_____
For nondairy, nonfortified sources:				+250
			Total:	_____

*Check food label for calcium content.

Figure 6-5.

Following the method outlined in figure 6-5, the total dietary intake for a person who consumes three or more dairy or highly calcium-fortified products (calcium-fortified citrus juice or hot cocoa), and adding 250 mg for trace sources of calcium in the diet, would be close to 1,200 mg per day—the desired intake for most middle-aged and older adults.

Many adults and even some children must follow certain dietary restrictions. In adults who are trying to reduce not only calories but also dietary fat and cholesterol, it may be difficult to modify the diet to obtain enough calcium. Certainly for those who drink orange or grapefruit juice regularly, switching to a calcium-fortified type is an easy modification. For the many individuals who would rather not spend time thinking about their diets, feel they are facing too many restrictions, or are for whatever reason still not getting at least three servings a day of calcium-dense foods, calcium supplements are fine. It is important to understand, though, that if calcium recommendations are met with food intake, no supplements are necessary. Many women, men, and even doctors are mistakenly suggesting calcium supplements in addition to calcium-rich diets. There is no evidence that this will benefit the skeleton. Even if you already have osteoporosis, healthy adults fifty-one years of age and over do not need to consume more than 1,200 or at most 1,500 mg of total calcium per day.

CALCIUM SUPPLEMENTS

There are many calcium supplements available. The most common chemical composition is calcium carbonate, but others include calcium citrates, calcium citrate malates, calcium hydroxyapatites, calcium lactates, and calcium gluconates. While the companies making these pills have marketing campaigns suggesting otherwise, in fact there is little evidence to indicate that one type of calcium supplement is better than another. The key ingredient in these supplements is the calcium, not the salt that is added to it (for instance, the carbonate, citrate, acetate, or gluconate). The major importance of knowing the brand of calcium is that the proportion of each pill that is calcium varies among the different calcium salts. In general, the calcium carbonates have the most calcium per pill (about 40 percent), whereas the calcium citrates have about 25 percent calcium per pill. The calcium lactates have only 10 percent calcium per pill. With some of these supplements, therefore, you must take more pills or bigger pills to get the same amount of calcium. To me, this is an undesirable feature of some supplements: Taking four to eight pills of a calcium supplement, rather than one or two, should in general be avoided. This is especially true considering that this is a general recommendation for all people to follow, not just those who have a disease.

Just as with foods, labeling on calcium supplement bottles can be extremely confusing. Sometimes the amount of calcium is actually given as the calcium salt complex. For example, a calcium carbonate supplement might be listed as supplying 1,000 mg of calcium carbonate, while the amount of true calcium or elemental calcium that it actually provides is only 400 mg. It is critical to look at the back label (small print) to determine the amount of elemental calcium provided by each pill. Another common mistake when reading supplement labels is that the amount of calcium supplied is often listed for multiple pills—for example, "two pills provide 630 mg of calcium." Many people miss the fact that in this case, one pill would provide only 315 mg of calcium.

It is useful to look for a USP (United States Pharmacopoeia) designation on the label of a calcium supplement. This symbol is added to products that have been voluntarily subjected to testing for solubility and purity. Many acceptable products have not been submitted to this testing. To guarantee that a product without a USP label will dissolve in the stomach, put the pill in a glass of clear vinegar to cover. It should dissolve within thirty minutes. If it doesn't, it may mean that it won't dissolve in your stomach, and an alternative preparation should be tried. The purity designation also indicates that the product has met standards for lead content. Lead is found throughout our environment, in our food, our drink, and the air we breathe. Likewise, calcium supplements can have a small amount of lead. The USP label indicates that the product meets acceptable standards for minute amounts of lead content. Furthermore, lead in calcium supplements is usually absorbed less well than lead from other ingested products, since calcium actually inhibits lead absorption.

Although some of the lay marketing literature states that certain calcium preparations are better absorbed than others, most studies suggest that the different salts that are available currently are absorbed equally well. Any apparent difference in calcium absorbability from different types of supplements is generally very minor. One important issue is how to take calcium supplements properly. For the most part, we recommend that people take calcium supplements with food, because the stomach acids produced in the process of digestion might improve the absorbability. Those people on calcium citrates need not take the supplements with food; in this case absorption does not depend on stomach acids. A special consideration in selecting calcium supplements is that, in the absence of stomach acid—a condition known as hypochlorhydria commonly found in elderly individuals—absorption may be reduced. Those individuals who are on high doses of acid-blocking medications for ulcer disease, acid reflux, or heartburn symptoms might also be less efficient at absorbing certain calcium supplements. Calcium citrate supplements may be preferable in these individuals.

In individuals whose diets provide less than 600 mg per day (as estimated using the method in figure 6-5), calcium supplements of more than 600 mg per day are necessary. We recommend separating the pills so that not all are taken at once. We actually absorb only a small fraction—20 to 30 percent—of the calcium in most supplements. (This is true of the calcium content in most foods also.) This small proportion of absorbed calcium is obviously taken into account when recommendations for total calcium intakes are developed. If we consume more than about 500 or 600 mg at a time, however, the absorption fraction becomes even less efficient, decreasing to below 20 or 30 percent. Thus, if you are taking two daily calcium supplement pills of greater than 500 to 600 mg, it's best to take them with two different meals.

While many Americans consume very little daily calcium, I also sometimes see patients who are consuming far too much. Those people who educate themselves about bone health often believe that if some is good, then more and more is better. One of my patients described her calcium regimen to me recently. She was eating calcium-fortified cereal with milk and drinking eight ounces of calcium-fortified juice each morning, having a cheese sandwich with milk for lunch each day, and eating a late-afternoon yogurt snack. She was also taking three 500 mg calcium pill supplements. The estimated calcium intake here is about 150 mg for half a cup of milk, 300 mg calcium from the cereal (taken from the nutritional facts on the cereal box), 400 mg from the two ounces of cheese on her sandwich, 300 mg from the lunchtime milk, 300 mg from yogurt, 250 mg from trace dietary calcium sources, plus 1,500 mg calcium from her supplements. A total of more than 3,200 mg per day! This is grossly excessive. There is no evidence confirming that excessive calcium has any benefit to bone. Instead, there may be a potential downside to consuming more than 2,500 mg per day. Most excessive calcium is excreted in the fecal matter, but it can produce abdominal discomfort with excessive gas and abdominal distension. Excessive calcium can also increase stomach acids and produce some heartburn-type symptoms. Furthermore, individuals who have kidney disease or a history of kidney stones should consult their doctor before starting calcium supplements. Lastly, preliminary data suggest a possible link between excessive chronic calcium consumption and prostate cancer.

A small group of individuals might absorb too much of the ingested calcium. This will be filtered into the urine and increase the amount of urine calcium. A potential side effect is an increase in the risk of kidney stones. In one very large observational study—the Nurses Health Study, a long-term investigation of more than seventy-two thousand nurses (see appendix A for a description)—there was no increase in risk of kidney stones in people who consumed large amounts of dietary calcium. In contrast, however, among people who took calcium supplements on an empty stomach, there was a slight increased risk of stone formation. Certainly, we should not take large amounts of calcium supplements if they are not needed. If you have had multiple kidney stones, you should ask your doctor for a twenty-four-hour urine calcium collection to make sure that your baseline calcium concentration is not elevated. Then the diet should be modified appropriately. If a calcium supplement is needed, it may be necessary to recheck urine calcium to make sure it does not become too high. One of the most important protective habits for anyone at risk for kidney stones is to make sure that fluid intake is substantial. A low fluid intake is one of the most important predictors of kidney stone risk.

INTESTINAL PROBLEMS AFFECTING CALCIUM INTAKES

Lactose Intolerance

Some individuals cannot absorb foods containing lactose, a type of sugar present in all dairy products. This may be a problem that develops in childhood or adulthood, and may present as a mild or severe problem. If you have symptoms of abdominal discomfort, distension, cramps, gas, and diarrhea after ingesting foods containing lactose (especially milk, cheese, and ice cream), you may be suffering from lactose intolerance. Individuals with this problem may be at particular risk of osteoporosis if they avoid many calcium-containing foods. If you have lactose intolerance, there is no reason for your calcium intake to be low, given the products currently available. Most individuals with lactose intolerance have no symptoms consuming dairy foods if consumed with lactase enzyme replacement available in pills, chewables, or powders. Many dairy foods are commercially available as lactose-reduced options where lactase has already been added. Calcium-fortified foods, non-dairy calcium sources, and calcium supplements should also suffice to overcome any dietary restrictions.

Malabsorption Syndromes

As for lactose intolerance, certain bowel diseases might make absorption of calcium, particularly from dairy products, difficult. A disorder called celiac disease or gluten-sensitive enteropathy, for example, can produce diarrhea and other abdominal/intestinal symptoms. This disorder, which may require severe dietary modifications such as avoiding all products containing gluten (barley, rye, oats, and wheat) may result in severe calcium malabsorption. It is thought that the ability to absorb calcium improves on a strict gluten-free diet. Even with complete avoidance of all gluten products, however, there may be some benefit to pushing calcium intake a bit higher in people with this condition (1,500 mg per day). Diseases such as inflammatory bowel conditions (ulcerative colitis and Crohn's disease) also often impair absorption of nutrients. Extra calcium and vitamin D are often warranted in these diseases as well. People who have had multiple abdominal surgeries, bowel resections, or ulcer surgeries might also benefit from pushing calcium intakes to 1,500 mg a day and increasing vitamin D consumption (see below).

ADJUSTING YOUR CALCIUM INTAKE

- Estimate your average daily calcium intake using figure 5 (checking food labels of fortified foods for calcium content).
- If your diet contains less than 1,200 mg per day, try to modify your diet to get more calcium.
- If you still fall short, take a calcium supplement to bring your total intake to at least 1,200 mg per day.
- Try to space your calcium-containing foods and/or supplements throughout the day.

VITAMIN D

Vitamin D is responsible for optimal calcium absorption and probably also has a direct effect on the skeleton. It is a fat-soluble vitamin, such that it can be stored for a long time in the body. There are only a few foods that naturally contain vitamin D. These include certain types of fish such as eel (which may be contained in sushi or sashimi products), fatty fishes (salmon, bluefish, and sardines), fish oil (cod liver oil), and eggs. The most common dietary source of vitamin D is fortified food, including milk, soy milk, rice milk, breakfast bars, and breakfast cereals.

When dietary sources of vitamin D are low, we can usually

compensate by making vitamin D through a precursor in the skin upon exposure to sunlight. The skin synthesis of vitamin D is reduced by wearing hats and clothing that covers most of the body, applying sunscreen, and by avoiding sun exposure altogether. All of these measures are important to protect the skin and reduce the risk of skin cancers. However, we may need to replace the vitamin D that the skin might have made with a vitamin. Most daily multivitamins contain about 400 International Units (IU) of vitamin D, which is adequate for most adults under the age of sixty-five.

For both women and men sixty-five and above, 700 to 800 IU of vitamin D per day is probably the optimal dose. Studies in older adults indicate that doses of vitamin D slightly higher than the RDI of 400 to 600 IU, in combination with 1,200 mg per day of calcium can reduce the risk of both hip and other fractures. A vitamin D intake of this level can easily be achieved by taking a daily multivitamin containing 400 IU per day and a calcium supplement containing 200 IU per tablet (taking one or two per day, as determined by dietary calcium intake) in addition to dietary sources. For those people who do not need any calcium supplements and/or do not want to take multivitamins, vitamin D can also be taken as an isolated supplement.

Vitamin D builds up in the body and is converted to active forms by both the liver and kidney. It is stored in fatty tissue; levels can be quite stable for days or weeks. Therefore, vitamin D does not need to be taken at the same time as calcium is taken. The upper limit for most healthy individuals is 2,000 IU per day. People with kidney or liver disease usually need vitamin D in different forms and doses than healthy women and men. People with other chronic illnesses may also need vitamin D. Those people already diagnosed with osteoporosis, particularly if it is severe, might need to have their vitamin D levels checked (see chapter 11), and pharmacologic doses of vitamin D are sometimes prescribed to return levels to a healthy point.

THE BARE BONES

- Adequate calories and protein are required for optimal skeletal health—but the most important building block for skeletal health is calcium. Vitamin D is also important.
- If you are above age fifty, you need at least 1,200 mg of calcium per day. This can be obtained by eating or drinking three or more calcium-rich foods or highly calcium-fortified foods each day.
- If it is very difficult for you to calculate your calcium intake and/or modify your diet, take a 600 mg calcium pill. The average intake in the United States is about 600 mg per day, so a 600 mg pill would fulfill the need for most individuals.
- Ideally, you should space calcium intake throughout the day.
- Certain foods, such as salt, protein, caffeine, fiber, and phytates, may have a modest influence on calcium absorption or calcium excretion. If you consume the recommended amount of calcium, you will overcome the modest effects of these other dietary products.
- Calcium supplements are available in tablet, chewable, or liquid forms. Some are constipating and produce excess gas. Others may produce slight queasiness.
- Most calcium supplements should be taken with food and plenty of fluid.

- If you are above age fifty, you should take a multivitamin or vitamin D supplement. More vitamin D is recommended for those sixty-five and above or those who have certain underlying diseases.

Chapter 7

Prevention Step Three: Exercise

Exercise is a critically important way to help prevent osteoporosis, maintain general good health, and avoid other chronic diseases such as cancer and vascular disease as well. This chapter reviews what happens when the body has no physical activity and discusses general concepts about what activities are required for optimal bone health. Tips on how to proceed with a gym-based exercise program are outlined, and other ideas about how to be successful with exercise routines are also offered. If you have any underlying medical problems, current or previous fractures, or have had a very sedentary lifestyle, ask your doctor for advice on getting started.

WHAT HAPPENS WITH INACTIVITY?

It is very clear, using the extreme example of outer space, that the complete void of gravitational pull or mechanical force on the skeleton can result in severe bone loss. Astronauts in space lose bone rapidly in the weight-bearing sites. In the heel, for example, up to 10 percent of bone mass can be lost within the first two to three months in space, and up to 20 percent can be lost within six months. This is one of the most important limitations to space travel, and the focus of several recent investigations has been to try to modify this risk. It is not yet known whether all or only some of this bone can be regained after returning to earth.

People who have been immobilized because of a disease, such as a severe stroke or spinal cord injury, usually lose a tremendous amount of bone in the year following the injury, primarily located in the part of the body that is immobilized. Illnesses that may involve reduced ambulation, such as multiple sclerosis, are also associated with loss of bone mass. Some studies indicate that even standing upright for as little as thirty minutes a day can prevent bone loss.

On the other end of the spectrum, however, in physically normal individuals, there are smaller differences. Physically active individuals generally have higher bone mass than inactive, sedentary individuals. This effect can be seen in young adults and adolescents where increased physical activity contributes to the attainment of a higher peak bone mass, and in older individuals where increased activity reduces the amount of bone loss. Still, in short-term exercise studies (one to three years in length), the magnitude of difference in bone mass between the exercising and nonexercising groups is small, averaging only about 1 percent per year. Of course, this can add up to substantial differences if the effect persists year after year.

Frequently, patients come to see me for follow-up after I've recommended an exercise program and they expect to see a big increase in their bone mass. Over less than three years, this is an unrealistic expectation. You cannot expect to gain a lot of bone, appreciable on bone density testing, after only a few years of even the most vigorous exercise regimen. Lifelong exercise, though, will ultimately have an impact on bone mass, falling risk, and fracture occurrence. Many observational studies of active versus inactive people show a reduced risk of hip and other fractures in the physically active group.

In the osteoporosis field, we often concentrate on bone, but it is equally important to consider the effects of exercise on muscle. Just as bone loss is an almost universal phenomenon with age, muscle wasting or loss of muscle mass is also universal with age. Muscle strength is directly proportionate to muscle mass, and reduced muscle strength is a strong risk factor for falling. Maintaining or improving muscle strength can help improve balance and coordination and thereby reduce the risk of falls. This is probably of particular importance in older individuals. Furthermore, exercise obviously has other major health benefits, such as protecting the heart and lungs and perhaps reducing the risk of certain cancers. It helps maintain healthy weight levels and may help prevent or treat mild depression. Maintaining good exercise habits is clearly one of the ways to help combat aging. It has struck me over the years of being in this field that the people who really seem to thrive in old age are those who are physically active, especially those who have been physically active their whole lives. Exercise is clearly one of the fountains of youth!

Although it's best if you start to exercise when you're young, it is never too late. You can find an appropriate and satisfying exercise regime at any age. Long periods of couch potato inactivity will end up costing you later in life—with detrimental effects on weight, diabetes, heart and other vascular disease, and cancer, general vigor, and endurance, as well as muscle mass, bone mass, and osteoporosis risk. A lifelong pattern of regular exercise will allow you to do what you want to do in retirement, to travel, and to enjoy your grandchildren. You'll look and feel 100 percent better!

THE EXERCISE PRESCRIPTION

All exercise regimens should be tailored to the individual's age and general health status and should consider the ability to maintain the program lifelong. The exact prescription for optimal attainment and maintenance of bone mass is unknown, but probably involves some combination of weight-bearing (on your feet) aerobic exercise and resistive muscle strengthening. Consult the sidebar on page 84 for general tips on exercising for osteoporosis prevention.

AEROBIC WEIGHT-BEARING PROGRAM FOR WELL PEOPLE

For people who are healthy and in decent physical condition, an aerobic weight-bearing exercise should ideally be performed three to five times a week to accomplish goals for both the skeleton and cardiovascular health. The new recommendations for optimal cardiovascular protection go even farther and suggest six days a week of aerobic exercise. In order to accomplish this goal, however, you can add in all of the exercise associated with normal daily activities—walking to stores, up and down stairs, and so forth. Simply walking twenty to thirty minutes a day, as a recreational activity or during the normal activities of daily living, has been associated with an improvement in bone health, and in general health, with associated decreases in mortality.

Other more vigorous weight-bearing aerobic activities include:

- Aerobic dance/calisthenics programs
- Cross-country skiing
- Dancing
- Treadmill for walking or jogging
- Exercise machines such as the stepper and elliptical walker (or moon walker)
- Jogging
- Racket sports (such as squash, tennis, racquetball)
- In-line skating
- Bicycling*
- Swimming**

*This may not be the most ideal bone-effective exercise, but can be used if enjoyed as part of the program, perhaps once or twice per week, in addition to doing a fully weight-bearing exercise two times per week.
**Despite the muscle strengthening, swimming's reduced-weight environment is an ineffective means of improving bone mass. As with cycling, however, if swimming is chosen for its overall health benefits and is enjoyable enough for an individual to keep it going, it should be done, but perhaps combined with a different weight-bearing activity on off-days—perhaps Monday and Friday swimming, Tuesday and Saturday jogging.

The extreme example of a weight-bearing exercise and its effect on bone is found in young women and girls who participate in high-impact exercises such as gymnastics. This sport involves a huge amount of jumping, especially from elevations (from uneven bars or balance beams, horses, vaults, and the like). This high-impact exercise seems to have a beneficial effect on bone mass during the time that the activity is being performed. Recently, results in studies of young children revealed that jumping rope or other jumping-type activities also have a significant positive effect on bone.

There is still no comprehensive consensus about the best bone-building exercise, but based on what we know right now, it might be reasonable for people who are healthy and motivated to add some form of jumping (high-impact loading) to their exercise routine. This is so incredibly vigorous, however, that usually it can only be part of the exercise regimen. It is unlikely that most adults would be able or would want to incorporate twenty to thirty minutes of jump roping three to five times a week. Furthermore, this may not be enjoyable enough for many people to keep going. In order to continue an exercise routine, it must be fun—or at least tolerable. No exercise routine will produce any long-term benefits unless it is continued. A reasonable suggestion might be to incorporate some jumping or jump roping into the exercise program, either with the rest of the aerobic regimen or as a separate activity at a different time of day or week. The optimal frequency (how many times per week to do it), duration (how long it should be done at each session), and intensity (how high should your feet and knees get and how fast should you jump) needed to get the best effects on bone are unknown.

EXERCISE RECOMMENDATIONS FOR SUFFERERS OF VERTEBRAL FRACTURES

For people who have some health impairments already, including prior osteoporosis-related fractures, especially those of the spine, high-impact exercise is not usually recommended. Compressive forces are generated in the spine during jumping and other jarring movements, and these may be too much for a spine already affected by vertebral compression fractures—or even with significant degenerative disk disease or arthritis unrelated to osteoporosis. Walking would be preferred to running in these patients because one foot is always on the ground during walking, whereas during running, both feet are temporarily in the air with the entire weight of the body landing on one foot.

Use caution or avoid:

- Bending forward with a rounded back
- Lifting
- Twisting of the torso
- Reaching far up and forward

All of these motions can produce forces in the vertebral bones that can facilitate further compression. Patients with new grandchildren may find it difficult to avoid picking up infants and toddlers. There may be such inherent benefits to these activities that they are worth the risk. They should be done very carefully, however. Any lifting at all must be done very carefully to avoid any forward bending or flexion of the torso; the back must be totally straight and the legs, particularly the thighs, must support the weight, with the knees bent to pick something up from the floor. Moreover, any significant pain occurring during any activity or exercise should make a person stop right away and should be a sign that this activity is not the right one for that individual.

Aerobic Exercise for Sufferers of Vertebral Fractures

- Ballroom dancing
- Elliptical or moon walker (a lower-impact form of the treadmill)
- Low-impact aerobic dance or calisthenics classes
- Rapid walking
- Stepper or stair-climbing machine

- Bicycling
- Swimming*

---

*Swimming may be particularly useful as an aerobic exercise in people who already have compression fractures because there is a lower risk of further injury. Muscle strengthening can be effectively accomplished with swimming, in addition to obtaining benefits with regard to cardiovascular training.

THE EXERCISE PRESCRIPTION: MUSCLE STRENGTHENING

Performing resistive exercise (using weights, weight machines, or just the weight of gravity) can augment muscle strength dramatically and help reduce the risk of falling and therefore fracturing. Comparable gains can be achieved with low-resistance, high-repetition programs as with high-resistance, lower-repetition programs. In general, these exercises should be initiated with the lowest possible weight load to make sure that injuries do not occur. Even in the long run, low weight or resistance may be preferable to high weight in order to avoid injury. Common injuries with weight-training programs are those that fall into the realm of soft-tissue injury, such as muscle strains or pulls and tendon inflammations or tendonitis. Although these injuries are not serious and almost always heal eventually, they can cause significant discomfort and temporary disability, may require health professional visits and medication, and certainly take people out of their exercise program for a while. Please consult the sidebar on page 84 for general tips on resistance-training programs.

It is important to concentrate on exercises for the large-muscle groups of the body, including the back muscles, shoulder and upper arm muscles, and pelvic/hip/thigh muscles. Depending on the exercises chosen for the aerobic weight-bearing program, some of these muscle groups are already being exercised. Certain aerobic activities, such as some dance routines (most prominently ballet), incorporate back muscle strengthening. For the back, you want to work on the muscles between the shoulder blades, the paraspinal muscles that lie along the spine on both sides, and the lower-back muscles, which stretch out to the side of the torso. The types of exercises that can strengthen these muscles include arching your back, push-ups, and moving your elbows back as if to touch each other behind your back. Whenever these exercises are done, it is important to keep the abdominal muscles tightened to avoid increasing the lumbar lordosis or keeping the lower back as flat as possible. Otherwise, low back pain might occur. (See figures 7-1 and 7-2.)

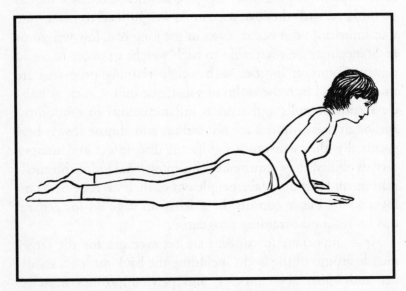

Figure 7-1: Movements to strengthen your back muscles.

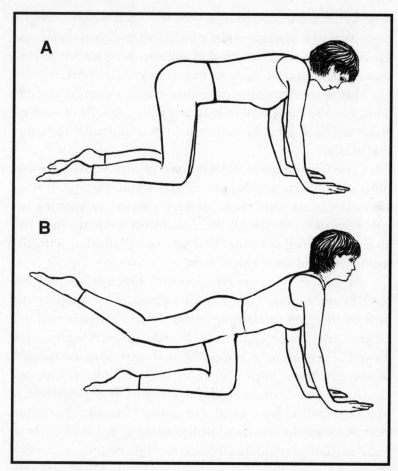

Figure 7-2: Movements to strengthen your back muscles.

It might be prudent, when initiating exercise, to consult with a physical therapist to get an idea of what is most important to add. Going through a circuit of exercise machines at a gym will usually hit all the important muscle groups. People can also be taught exercises to do at home with free hand weights, weights that attach to wrists and ankles with Velcro and elastic bands. Alternately, a good old-fashioned calisthenics program where exercises are done against the force of gravity will also work.

Muscle-strengthening programs, which are not that strenuous, can also be helpful in reducing falling risk. Almost all exercise regimens have been shown to have potential to reduce risk of falls.

• Tai Chi, an ancient Asian form of exercise that involves slow, graceful arm and leg movements while standing, is not a vigorous exercise but might be very effective at training dynamic balance. Almost all the movements are performed balancing on one leg at a time. This may be a particularly effective regimen for reducing risk of falls.

• Pilates exercises are very popular currently. This program can be done at home on a mat with a book or videotape or can be done in a gym specializing in this form of exercise, with specialized equipment (Reformer, Wunda Chair, Cadillac, and Tower). These exercises are excellent at increasing the strength of the core muscles of the spine, neck, abdomen, hip, and thigh as well as increasing their flexibility. It is purported to produce lean and long muscles in contrast to bulky short muscles. Some of the exercises involve some spinal flexion, however, so if this program appeals to you, consult a physical therapist about which exercises to avoid or modify. Most of the program is probably excellent for osteoporosis prevention.

• Yoga is a set of different exercise routines involving body poses usually held for some time and concentrating on strength, balance, and flexibility as well as relaxation. There are many different types of yoga, including ashtanga, bikram, hatha, integral, iyengar, jivamukti-style, Kali Ray Tri Yoga, kripalu, kundalini, power yoga, sivananda, svaroopa, viniyoga, white lotus, and others. Some are more vigorous than others, many concentrate on breathing, and some include chanting. There are some poses and postures that put a lot of compressive force on the spine and others that put the spine into flexion. These postures can easily be avoided in any yoga routine while you still get the benefits of these programs.

IMPORTANT EXERCISE FACTS

- There may be an advantage to performing different exercises on different days with different muscles being worked. In the long run, this may facilitate optimal bone and muscle benefits while reducing risks of injury.
- During childhood and adolescence, when bones are still growing in length, exercise might not only improve bone mass but also make bones larger, an effect that can improve strength of bone dramatically. Nevertheless, exercise can improve bone mass and strength in people at any age.
- It appears that with any exercise program, as soon as you stop, the skeletal benefits wane and ultimately disappear. Weight lifters have elevated bone mass during their lifting years, but within ten years of discontinuing the sport they are no different than their non-weight-lifting peers.
- Any exercise is better than none. You shouldn't feel discouraged if you can work in an exercise routine only once or twice a week; this is a good start and could really make a difference. Once this becomes habit, it may be possible to extend it. Even bursts of activity such as cleaning the house once a week and running up and down stairs with multiple loads of laundry will keep you more fit, bone and otherwise, than you would be if totally sedentary.

- Start slowly; it is unrealistic to expect a previously sedentary fifty-year-old to be able to jog three miles three times a week. Ultimately that may happen if you begin with walking and slowly incorporate a few minutes of jogging each session, and thus increase the amount over months or years.
- Vary the exercise activities to make them more fun.
- Try to exercise with family members or friends to add a social element to it.
- Incorporate physical activity into leisure time as much as possible.
- Try to choose activities you enjoy so that they can become lifelong habits.
- It is generally accepted that stretching before and after exercise is beneficial, though good evidence that this is true is lacking. Injuries can occur when people stretch too aggressively. Perhaps most important is starting the exercise slowly until the involved muscles warm up.

EXERCISE TIPS FOR MANAGEMENT OF OSTEOPOROSIS

General

- **Combine an aerobic exercise, done while standing, with a general muscle-strengthening program. Those people who cannot do a standing (weight-bearing) exercise will still benefit from exercise done while sitting or lying down.**
- **Start very slowly. You are trying to create lifelong habits. No program is effective in the long term if you don't keep doing it.**

- Any exercise is better than none.
- Any discomfort beyond some muscle soreness should prompt you to stop that exercise and ask for advice.

Weight-Bearing Aerobic Program

- Include walking or jogging, dancing, racquet sports, aerobics.
- Include exercise machines such as a treadmill, elliptical walker, stepper or stairclimbing machine, cross-country ski machine. If you are using exercise machines:
  - Start very slowly.
  - You can combine the use of more than one machine, but your total duration should usually not exceed forty-five to sixty minutes.
  - If you've been sedentary, start with five to ten minutes of exercise at very slow speed.
  - Slowly increase the duration of exercise to a total of about thirty minutes, adding about one or two minutes every week or two.
  - Once a duration of thirty minutes is reached, increase your speed very slowly, with small changes at most every one to two weeks.

Muscle-strengthening Program

Concentrate on the large muscles of the back, shoulder and upper arms, buttocks, pelvis, hips, and upper legs. With gym equipment or exercise machines:

- It's generally wise to avoid more than two machines or devices for the same area.
- Start with one set of three to twelve repetitions, depending on your baseline strength.
- Start with no added weight.
- Increase the number of repetitions to a maximum of fifteen.
- Increase the weight by the smallest possible increment (you may need to decrease your repetitions by a few at first when the weight is added).
- Do not add weight more than once every two weeks.
- Add a second set of repetitions if all of the above is accomplished.

- For the back:
  - Gravitron or other machines allowing pull-ups and bar dips
  - Back extension machines
  - Sitting row
  - Latissimus pull-downs

- For the upper arms:
  - Gravitron or other machines allowing pull-ups and bar dips
  - Latissimus pull-downs
  - Bench press/arm press

- For the buttocks:
  - Elliptical walker backward (one minute)

- Stair-climbing machine forward or backward
- Ankle attachment to universal gym with leg extension
- Leg press

- For the pelvis/hips:
  - Ankle attachment to universal gym with hip flexion and hip abduction
  - Leg abductor and adductor machines

- For the upper legs:
  - Quadriceps (knee extension) machine
  - Hamstrings (knee flexion) machine
  - Leg press
  - Thigh abductor and adductor machines

At home, try the following:

- Back arches while lying on your abdomen with your arms at your sides or folded under your chin.
- Modified standing push-ups standing twelve inches away from the wall.
- On your hands and knees, lift one leg upward with your back arched and hold for five seconds.
- Standing and holding on to a chair, lift one leg straight behind you and hold for five seconds.
- Standing and holding on to a chair, lift one leg straight out to the side with your toes forward.

- Add Thera-Bands (elastic bands) for back muscle and leg strengthening.
- Video or television classes can offer good general muscle-strengthening programs. See appendix B for Web sites containing more information; start with the NOF.

THE BARE BONES

- Physical inactivity results in bone loss.
- Ask your doctor for a referral to a physical therapist for help in getting started if you have underlying medical problems or have had a very sedentary lifestyle.
- It is important to start any exercise program slowly for short periods of time to avoid injury.
- The best exercise for bone is a combination of weight-bearing aerobic exercise and resistance training. Weight-bearing exercise can be done in the gym, at home (with machines or aerobic exercise tapes), outdoors (jogging, in-line skating), or as part of a recreation program (tennis, racquetball, dancing). Resistance training can be done in a gym, with free weights, weights that strap on to ankles and wrists and elastic bands, or using exercise tapes with calisthenics done against gravity.
- You must maintain good postural alignment during exercise to avoid injury and optimize benefits.
- Pick an exercise that is enjoyable; vary it to keep it interesting; do it with a buddy to help make it more fun and keep going.
- Exercise will provide long-term benefits only if it is continued.

Chapter 8

Prevention Step Four:
Supplements and Vitamins?

This chapter briefly outlines our current knowledge about several over-the-counter vitamins and supplements, including boron, zinc, copper, manganese, magnesium, soy products and ipriflavene, and vitamins A, B, C, and K (listed in alphabetical order). The optimal level of each of these nutrients is unknown, but most medical professionals believe that a good basic diet, with lots of fruits and vegetables and whole grains, should supply whatever is necessary. A basic daily multivitamin can provide additional nutrients. Many have advocated additional supplemental pills containing these and other substances as important for bone and other health concerns. The evidence, however, that specific supplements (other than calcium and vitamin D) are needed or even beneficial to the skeleton in the majority of healthy individuals is lacking. Furthermore, there may be deleterious effects associated with some of these products. One very important distinction between calcium and these other nutrients is that a large proportion of the skeleton is actually calcium. This is not true of the other nutrients; for bone health, therefore, it is less likely that these other nutrients would be required in large doses.

BORON

Boron is a chemical element found in nature and used in home products as a washing powder. Boron has no known function in humans and is not recognized as an essential nutrient. Dietary sources of boron include water, nuts, peanut butter, milk, prune and grape juices, wine, dried beans, potatoes, coffee, milk, and apples. There is no currently recommended daily intake established for boron. One laboratory has reported an improvement in calcium metabolism in postmenopausal women given boron supplements (3 mg per day). However, other laboratories have not been able to reproduce those findings. *Thus, it is not recommended to take supplemental boron.*

COPPER

A healthy diet and/or a daily multivitamin will provide adequate copper intake. This mineral is important for normal bone metabolism; the RDA for adults is 900 mcg per day. *Dietary sources include seafood, nuts, seeds, cereals, whole grains, cocoa, and organ meats.*

MANGANESE

This mineral is needed for normal bone metabolism. Adequate intakes are 1.8 mg per day in women and slightly higher in men (2.3 mg per day). *Dietary sources include nuts, vegetables, tea, whole grains, and drinking water.* The requirements can be easily met by a typical U.S. or vegetarian diet. Although manganese is available in a variety of supplements, it is not needed or recommended for bone health.

MAGNESIUM

Magnesium is a mineral element widely distributed in nature and an important constituent of all cells. Magnesium is important for normal calcium balance. The current RDA for women is 320 mg per day; for men, it is 420 mg. The best dietary sources of magnesium include dark green vegetables, whole grains, bananas, nuts, and seeds. Refined foods have very low magnesium content. When magnesium levels in the blood and other tissues of humans are low, the mechanisms for regulating bone remodeling and for controlling blood calcium do not function correctly. There is no evidence that deficiency sufficient to disrupt calcium regulation in this way ever occurs at typical magnesium intakes in otherwise healthy individuals. Moreover, several studies have shown clearly that, in individuals consuming typical U.S. diets, magnesium is not needed for normal calcium absorption, and magnesium supplements do not influence bone tissue maintenance. Although magnesium is often added to calcium supplements, most individuals do not need additional magnesium for bone health.

Results of the observational arm (see appendix A for an explanation) of the Women's Health Initiative were recently presented. This is a study of more than ninety-three thousand healthy postmenopausal women. The relationship between bone density and fracture occurrence was assessed in relationship to total magnesium intake, including both diet and supplements. Results of the analysis indicated that those women who had the highest magnesium intakes had a slightly higher bone density; however, this group of women also had the highest risk of fracture occurrence. Moreover, even in women with the lowest magnesium intakes, there was no increase in the risk of fracture.

Patients who have malabsorption syndromes (diseases causing difficulty processing, digesting, and assimilating nutrients from foods) may develop significant magnesium deficiency. These exceptions include people with bowel diseases such as Crohn's disease, celiac disease, or any chronic diarrheal illness; alcoholics; diabetics; and people who have recently received chemotherapy or are on other medications that might produce magnesium wasting. When the underlying disorder is controlled by medication or diet, there still may be some residual magnesium deficiency, which could interfere with bone health. Under such circumstances magnesium deficiency may be diagnosed on a blood test and magnesium supplements may be required.

Some people find that calcium supplements can be constipating. In those individuals, choosing a calcium supplement that also supplies magnesium can be beneficial to help regulate bowel function. However, it may be relatively easy to intake magnesium beyond the tolerable upper limit of 350 mg/day of supplemental magnesium. Above this level, adverse effects might occur even in healthy individuals.

In people with kidney disease, magnesium supplements should be avoided, and in otherwise healthy individuals magnesium supplements are not required.

OMEGA-3 FATTY ACIDS

Omega-3 fatty acids are present in both certain plant sources (lignans contained in soybeans, flaxseed, and walnuts) as well as animal sources (from fatty fish such as salmon, mackerel, and sardines). Laboratory studies in bone cells and animal research suggest that these compounds might produce some beneficial effect on bone; there are no human studies to confirm this, however. Vegetable sources may be preferable to fish sources to avoid associated high intakes of vitamin A (see below).

PHYTOESTROGENS

Phytoestrogens are estrogenic substances derived from plant sources. Dietary products such as soy foods, chickpeas and other legumes, and red clover contain phytoestrogens, which may have some health-promoting effects. Epidemiologic evidence has shown a low prevalence of both heart disease and breast cancer in areas such as Southeast Asia where there is a high consumption of soy foods. An accumulating body of evidence suggests that these compounds may be similar to the SERM drugs (see chapter 15), meaning they have some positive estrogenlike actions on bone metabolism and bone mass of modest magnitude.

Studies in monkeys have shown that phytoestrogens from soy products, called isoflavones, specifically genistein and daidzein, inhibit bone loss. Studies in the monkey also indicate that phytoestrogens can improve plasma lipoproteins, decrease atherosclerosis, and maintain coronary artery vasodilation.

There are also a few small clinical trials in postmenopausal women suggesting that phytoestrogens can help maintain bone mass and reduce the incidence and severity of menopause-related hot flashes when compared to placebo. Not all of the latter studies are consistent, however, with some indicating no effect. Several small human studies indicate that isoflavones might decrease total cholesterol and LDL cholesterol (the detrimental type) and perhaps even reduce blood pressure slightly. Unlike animal estrogens (but similar to raloxifene), phytoestrogens do not appear to stimulate the uterus or breast, although clinical trial data evaluating these outcomes, and the effects of phytoestrogens on cardiovascular disease, and fractures are all lacking.

Clearly, these compounds should be studied further to elucidate their effects on various organ systems. The effects of high doses easily obtained in pill form may differ from those of the lower doses that can be consumed in the diet, and their safety particularly for the breast and uterus have not been determined. *While it may be reasonable at this time, with limited information, to recommend using moderate amounts of soy products in the diet, it is not recommended that people consume isoflavone-derivative pills, particularly for a prolonged period of time, where high doses of purified isoflavones can easily be ingested.*

IPRIFLAVONE

Ipriflavone is a synthetic derivative of isoflavones, available over the counter without a doctor's prescription. It is considered a dietary supplement and is touted by its manufacturers for use in management of osteoporosis. Studies using rats have shown a preservation of bone tissue when the rats were given ipriflavone. Several small studies evaluating ipriflavone in humans indicated that it could help maintain bone mass in postmenopausal women. However, the definitive study performed on more than four hundred women with osteoporosis indicated that ipriflavone does not improve bone density or bone turnover; nor does it reduce the occurrence of vertebral fractures. Moreover, it actually produced a reduction in the number of lymphocytes in a significant number of women, some of whom had not returned to normal two years after stopping the medicine. *Therefore, ipriflavone is not recommended and might in fact be dangerous.*

VITAMIN A

Vitamin A is an essential fat-soluble vitamin required for vision, growth, and immune function. It also plays a role in bone remodeling. Vitamin A is actually a family of substances that includes retinol (preformed vitamin A) and carotenoids, which can be converted to vitamin A. Retinol, the most abundant form, is found in foods of animal origin such as organ meats, fish and fish oils, egg yolks, fortified milk, and breakfast cereals and bars. Carotenoids including beta-carotene are present in dark green and orange fruits and vegetables. The proportion of the retinol and beta-carotene contents of both foods and vitamin supplements differ, and the efficiency with which these substances are converted to vitamin A differs; therefore, it is difficult to calculate vitamin A intakes.

A recent finding from the Nurses Health Study—an observational study of more than 72,000 female nurses—showed that high intakes of vitamin A, specifically the retinol component of vitamin A, may be associated with an elevated risk of having a hip fracture. Specifically, hip fracture rates were doubled in women who had retinol intakes of more than 2,000 mcg per day compared to women with intakes less than 500 mcg per day. This did not seem to be true of the beta-carotene form of vitamin A, which even in high doses was not associated with increased hip fracture risk.

For optimal skeletal health, it may be prudent to avoid overconsumption of retinol from concentrated sources such as liver and fish oils and supplements; however, liberal amounts of vitamin-A-containing fruits and vegetables should be consumed. Most multivitamins and supplements contain a combination of the retinol and carotene forms of vitamin A. Certain multivitamins are actually changing formulation as a result of the recent data. The recommended dietary allowance for total vitamin A is 700 RAE (Retinol Activity Equivalents) (2,300 IU) per day for women, and 900 RAE (3,000 IU) per day for men. The tolerable upper limit for retinol is 3,000 RAE (10,000 IU) per day while there is no upper limit for beta-carotene. *It is clear that people should not take extra amounts of vitamin A in supplements in the hope of improving their bone health.*

VITAMIN B (FOLIC ACID, VITAMIN B$_{12}$, VITAMIN B$_6$)

Recent clinical trials of B vitamin complexes have indicated that B vitamins can reduce the levels of a variety of substances present in the blood associated with heart disease. Folic acid is also specifically recommended for pregnant women to reduce the risk of spinal cord malformations and nervous system defects such as spina bifida. Most recently, the American Medical Association has come out with a recommendation that most or all adults should be taking a multivitamin containing folic acid, vitamin B$_{12}$, and vitamin B$_6$. There are few data evaluating the influence of the B vitamins on bone health. *Thus, a one-a-day multivitamin should probably be taken for a variety of reasons, but no additional vitamin B supplements should be taken for the purpose of improving bone health.*

VITAMIN C

Vitamin C is an essential vitamin for the production of normal skin and bone. This vitamin is found in high concentrations in citrus fruit and juices, green leafy vegetables, tomatoes, broccoli, peppers, and potatoes. The RDA is 75 mg/day for women and 90 mg/day for men, easily achievable by diet alone. Observational studies show a possible positive relationship between vitamin C intake and bone mass, but there are no controlled clinical trials (see appendix A) showing that vitamin C supplementation can improve bone mass or reduce fractures. *A high intake of fruits and vegetables will likely provide enough vitamin C for bone health. Additional ingestion of vitamin C supplements for osteoporosis prevention or treatment cannot be endorsed at this time.*

VITAMIN K

Vitamin K is a nutrient needed by the body to form the protein compounds involved in blood coagulation as well as specialized proteins in tissues throughout the body, including bone. Some observational studies have found that women with higher vitamin K intakes have higher bone densities and lower rates of fracture. This vitamin can be found in highest concentration in dark green leafy vegetables and vegetable oils such as soybean, canola, and olive oil. The AI (Adequate Intake) for vitamin K is 90 mcg for women and 120 mcg for men daily. A healthy well-balanced diet high in vegetables is likely to provide adequate vitamin K. Since vitamin K is fat-soluble, individuals with malabsorption can become deficient. These people should discuss whether supplementation is needed. Although there are a few small studies looking at vitamin K supplementation indicating that it might have some protective effect on bone, *at this time there is insufficient evidence to recommend that women take vitamin K supplements.* If you are on blood-thinning medication, your doctor may advise you to avoid high intakes of vitamin K.

ZINC

Zinc is another mineral that may be required in minute quantities for healthy bone metabolism. Recommended intakes are 8 mg per day for women and 11 mg per day for men. Dietary sources of zinc include fortified cereals, eggs, dairy foods, nuts, red meat, peas, and some seafood. Zinc deficiency is uncommon in healthy people but may occur and require treatment in those with malabsorption syndromes. *People who have kidney disease must be careful not to take any zinc supplements. A healthy diet and/or a daily multivitamin will supply adequate zinc.*

THE BARE BONES

- More than five servings a day of fruits and vegetables will meet the requirements for many nutrients and improve skeletal health.
- A daily multivitamin can provide additional minerals and vitamins to ensure that all of the skeleton's needs are met. The use of a multivitamin may have other health benefits with respect to heart disease and cancer. Daily multivitamins are safe and inexpensive. Look for vitamins that contain vitamin A primarily from beta-carotene, not retinol.
- There are insufficient data to recommend specific supplementation with any one mineral or vitamin or other nutri-

ents (aside from calcium or vitamin D) for osteoporosis prevention or treatment in otherwise healthy individuals at this time.

- If you have gastrointestinal disease or malabsorption, you should ask your doctor about specific supplementation with other nutrients, such as magnesium, zinc, and vitamin K.

- Phytoestrogens in soy food products and derivatives may be overall healthful to add to our diets, but purified isoflavone derivatives have not been studied well enough to be guaranteed of safety to breast or other organ systems, and therefore should be discouraged, particularly for long-term use. Ipriflavone does not produce any benefit to bone health and may be unhealthy in other ways. *Ipriflavone should not be taken.*

Part III

DIAGNOSING
OSTEOPOROSIS

Chapter 9

Are You at Risk?

The suggestions in part II of this book concerning osteoporosis prevention are universal preventive measures. All individuals, young and old, should follow them, whether or not there is a specific risk for osteoporosis. The genetic factors that confer osteoporosis risk may be so dominant, however, that even people who follow bone-healthy lifestyle measures from childhood may still develop osteoporosis. Certain diseases increase risk and not beginning preventive measures early enough in life might also predispose toward development of osteoporosis. The only way to determine if you have osteoporosis or are at high risk of developing osteoporosis is to get a bone density test. But I don't mean to suggest that no matter who or how old you are, you should immediately run out for a test. This chapter discusses the risk factors, including age, body weight, prior fracture history, family history of fractures, smoking, and chronic diseases, which should alert you to the possibility that you might have osteoporosis.

While it may seem to make sense to determine your bone density during youth at the time at which peak bone mass has been acquired, since no medical interventions are currently available at this stage of life, in general bone mass should not be measured. There are of course a few exceptions to this principle, such as osteoporosis as a result of steroid treatment (see chapter 23). At some point in the future when a medication or other intervention is developed that can actually build bone mass during this early period of life, then a bone density test might be warranted during youth. At that point, at least there would be some action that could be taken if the bone density result is not favorable. As of this writing, however, there are no bone-building drugs for this phase of life. Instead, all of the medications we now have are those that lower bone turnover (which is already low at this phase of life) and prevent bone loss, with the one exception of PTH, a bone-building treatment for postmenopausal women and men with severe osteoporosis. During youth, optimal nutrition, regular exercise, and healthy lifestyle choices can help you attain your genetically determined peak bone mass. If you, any young woman you know, or your own children are not involved in an exercise program, let me remind you that the threat of osteoporosis is one more reason to take care of yourself *now!*

AGE

In part as a result of the dramatic increase in occurrence of osteoporosis-related fractures with advancing age, and the type of medications that are now available to treat osteoporosis, one of the most effective times to perform bone density testing is in women aged sixty-five and older. Our current health care system will reimburse the vast majority of these tests in this age group. Anyone who has not yet had a bone density test by this age should have the test done. This recommendation is for women only. We have not yet developed good guidelines for determining who among men should have the bone density test. It is likely that we will recommend routine testing at a later age in men, because their risk of osteoporosis is somewhat lower than in women. In fact, the currently available guidelines refer specifically to Caucasian women. Women of other ethnicities may have different underlying risks of fracture. Women of Asian and Hispanic descent probably have risks similar to those of the Caucasian woman. Risks in African American women are somewhat lower, perhaps similar to those in Caucasian men, whereas the risk in African American men is even lower. In lieu of any other specific recommendations for women of non-Caucasian descent, it is reasonable to apply the same screening and treatment principles to these women as for Caucasians. The remainder of this chapter refers to women.

The time of menopause is also a very appropriate one to evaluate risk of osteoporosis. At this stage of life, many chronic diseases begin to increase in frequency, including heart disease and cancer as well as osteoporosis. The dramatic reduction in estrogen levels at menopause is associated with dramatic reductions in bone mass. Therefore, a bone density test to determine whether medication is needed makes tremendous sense at this stage. It is my professional opinion and personal belief that at menopause, all women should get a bone density test. This is a noninvasive, zero-risk procedure that is our only way to definitely determine osteoporosis risk and, most importantly, to determine who needs medication and who does not, before fractures occur. Because of cost concerns, however, it is difficult to recommend the test as a universal public health measure at menopause. Instead, we have identified a set of risk factors, thought to be independent of bone mass as predictors of fracture risk. We have used these risk factors to determine which women should get a bone density test at the time of menopause, prior to the age of sixty-five. If you are below the Medicare age, you should check with your insurance about coverage for bone density tests. Many health maintenance organizations (HMOs) and private insurers will pay for a screening test in women at the time of menopause.

ADULTHOOD FRACTURES WITH LITTLE TRAUMA

Many adulthood fractures (occurring at age thirty-five or later) that occur in the absence of major trauma can be attributed at least in part to osteoporosis. In contrast, a bad automobile accident or an accident in which a pedestrian is hit by a car or motorcycle obviously could be enough to break bones in even the healthiest, largest person with the strongest skeleton. Also, many athletic injuries that occur during high-speed falls—during skiing, for example—would not qualify as fractures related to osteoporosis. Falling off something elevated above ground, such as a ladder, and fracturing a bone may not be a sign of osteoporosis. Some have argued that even many of these trauma-induced fractures may be attributed in part to osteoporosis. This is debatable depending on the level of trauma.

But most fractures that occur from routine falls while standing are a possible sign that osteoporosis or reduced bone mass might be present. Having one or more of these fractures in your personal history should make you get an earlier bone density test (at the time of menopause or perimenopause, usually late forties to early fifties).

A history of spine or hip fracture is a particularly important predictor of future fracture frequency. Almost every single individual who has had one of these fractures in the absence of major trauma should take a medication for osteoporosis, even if bone density results are not particularly low (see part IV for treatment recommendations).

FAMILY HISTORY OF OSTEOPOROSIS-RELATED FRACTURES

Another extremely important risk factor that would warrant an individual having an earlier bone density test is a family history of osteoporosis or osteoporotic fracture. A maternal history of hip fracture may be the most convincing of the historical factors, but probably any maternal history of fracture would be a risk factor for the individual. It is also important to ask about the family history in the father, any aunts, uncles, grandparents, or siblings. If you ask the question, "Did your mother's sister ever have osteoporosis?" the answer will usually be no. Osteoporosis was rarely diagnosed as a disease before the late 1980s or even early 1990s, primarily because the noninvasive, simple way to diagnose it was not readily available until that time. Also, most people do not realize that a fracture that occurs in a fall is often an osteoporotic fracture. They usually attribute the fracture to trauma. Another clue to the presence of osteoporosis in a family member might be a person who developed a very hunched-over or stooped posture and lost a lot of height. Not everyone who loses height has significant osteoporosis. People lose height because of degenerative disk disease and progression of scoliosis, in addition to vertebral compression fractures. Furthermore, not everyone who develops the classic dowager's hump has vertebral osteoporosis. Some of this abnormal posture probably relates to other degenerative diseases. There are also some rare genetic diseases causing problems with some of the vertebral bones that are distinct from osteoporosis (two examples are Scheuermann's disease and juvenile kyphosis). Nevertheless, having a family member who lost more than two inches of height or whose posture became very stooped might be a clue toward a genetic predisposition toward developing osteoporosis. Having a family member who experienced a wrist, hip, leg, arm, or known spine fracture in a fall is also a clue to a possible genetic predisposition toward osteoporosis.

LOW BODY WEIGHT

Women who weigh less than 127 pounds are also at higher risk for osteoporosis and should have an earlier bone density test. This is a very general statement, because of course short women who weigh less than 127 pounds may not actually be so thin. Determining how thin you are at a certain weight must take into account your height. Nevertheless, the calculation of reduced body fat, which takes into account both height and weight, is not really any more predictive of risk of osteoporosis than is weight itself, so we use a weight cutoff of 127 pounds to indicate those who are at elevated risk for fracture.

Weight is a determinant of bone density but may also be mechanically protective. Extra weight can put an extra daily load on bones to stimulate bone formation, similar to what exercise does. Extra weight can also facilitate production of estrogens from fatty tissue. This is one of the only health areas where a little extra weight actually does something beneficial.

SMOKING

Smoking is such an important risk factor for osteoporosis that anyone who smokes should have a bone density test right at the time of menopause. Recent quitters should also have an earlier bone density assessment, although people with a remote smoking history are probably back to baseline risk; they would not require an earlier bone density test.

CHRONIC DISEASES

Having a disease that increases the risk of osteoporosis, such as rheumatoid arthritis or inflammatory bowel disease, should motivate a woman to speak to her doctor about having an earlier bone density test (see chapter 10). Chronic or frequent use of medications such as steroids or thyroid hormone without regular blood test monitoring would also make us recommend a bone density test at the time of menopause. Diseases that limit mobility and increase the risk of falling and osteoporosis, such as multiple sclerosis and Parkinson's disease, should also mandate earlier testing for osteoporosis.

OTHER RISK FACTORS FOR OSTEOPOROSIS

There are many other risk factors for osteoporosis. In many cases, it is legitimate to obtain a bone density test at the time of menopause if any of these factors is present. The issue of whether insurance companies will reimburse for the test in all of these cases sometimes gets in the way of better judgment. Again, if cost were not an issue at all, I think it would be advisable for all women to get a bone density measurement at menopause.

BONE QUALITY

Factors such as the geometry of bone, and the underlying microscopic architecture of bone, are clearly important to bone strength. How much mineral there is in the existing bone is another important qualitative factor. The number of healthy cells living in a piece of bone may be another determinant of bone quality and ultimate bone strength. These factors may add to the ability to predict an individual's likelihood of having a fracture. Right now we can't measure these things, but probably within the next five years, we'll be able to.

THE BARE BONES

- You may be at risk for osteoporosis if you have one or more of the following risk factors:
  - Advanced age
  - Caucasian, Asian, or Hispanic race
  - Prior history of nonchildhood fracture, especially spine or hip fracture (consider possible evidence of vertebral fracture such as height loss of more than two inches, dowager's hump, or chronic back pain)
  - Family history of fracture
  - Low body weight
  - Early menopause or very irregular or infrequent menstrual periods when young
  - Smoking
  - Excessive alcohol consumption
  - Chronic diseases such as rheumatoid arthritis, celiac disease or malabsorption
  - Use of medications such as steroids, high doses of thyroid hormone, or antiseizure medication
  - Low testosterone in men

- The only way to accurately determine your risk of osteoporosis-related fracture prior to the occurrence of a fracture is to have a bone density test.

- All women should have a bone density test at least by the age of sixty-five, or at the age of menopause if there are clinical risk factors present. If your insurance covers bone density testing for all women at menopause or if you are willing to pay for the test yourself, you should get it done even in the absence of clinical risk factors.

- In the future, we may be able to measure other qualitative abnormalities in bone to help refine the ability to determine which people are most likely to fracture.

Chapter 10

Getting Tested: Measuring and Reporting Bone Mass

Once you have determined that a bone density test is needed or recommended (see chapter 9), you need to figure out what test to have. There are several types of bone density measuring devices. Some of these may be present in doctors' offices, mobile units, or health fairs and malls, and others are found usually only in radiology centers or hospitals. It's important to understand the advantages and disadvantages of the different measurement techniques.

CENTRAL DUAL X-RAY ABSORPTIOMETRY

The best method for determining your bone density is the central dual X-ray absorptiometry technique (central DXA). This machine can be found in certain mobile van units, but is most often located in hospitals and radiology centers. On occasion, these machines are also found in high-volume medical practices in private offices. Anyone living in an urban or suburban area will have access to one of these machines.

The central DXA machine looks like a hospital stretcher

with the bottom filled in. It has a thin padded table on top, a movable arm above, and is attached to a computer. The bottom part has an X-ray device built into it. A person having bone density measured can be fully clothed, but should not have any metal zippers or brassiere fasteners overlying the back. The test is totally noninvasive and requires no needles or dyes. The person lies on the padded table, and X rays come from underneath. There are X rays of two different energies, which are absorbed by the body and bones in different amounts. The amount of radiation that is subsequently picked up by the movable arm above the body is used to calculate how much bone and how much soft tissue (muscle or fat) is there.

The areas most often measured using central DXA are the hip and spine. With modern machines, the measurement usually only takes five to ten minutes. The forearm/wrist and total body are also sometimes measured. The hip DXA measurement is the single best way to determine bone density because it predicts the risk of hip fracture better than any other single measurement, and it predicts the risk of all other fractures as well as any other single measurement.

The spine DXA is also usually measured at the same time as the hip DXA, for the same cost. Often, in people of advancing age, the spine measurement has a lot of artifact from scoliosis, arthritis, degenerative disk disease, compressions of vertebral bones, or sometimes from calcifications in the aorta, the large artery that overlies the spine. Therefore, it might not be a very accurate measurement in older individuals. At bone density testing centers where there is good quality control, the interpreter will look at the spine image and bone density results for the individual spine bones measured. If there is an apparent compression or bone spur overlying one of the bones, the reader might exclude that bone and obtain a truer bone density result than if all the vertebral bones are included. Many times, I have seen patients who have had their bone densities misinterpreted. A person's bone mass can look normal in the spine if one or two of the bones are substantially falsely elevated, whereas if those one or two vertebrae are excluded by a careful reader, the person might be diagnosed with osteoporosis.

In contrast to the spine measurement, arthritis or other common artifacts rarely affect the hip bone mineral density (BMD) measurement. Therefore, in people sixty-five years of age and above, the hip DXA measurement should be considered more accurate than the spine measurement. In other words, if there is a low hip value and normal or high spine value, the hip value should be the one used to gauge need for treatment.

Those individuals with one high and one low bone density measure might have an intermediate risk of all fractures, compared to those for whom both measures are low. Thus more people at slightly lower risk of fracture might end up being treated if the lowest measurement of several is used to determine whether treatment is indicated. This makes good clinical sense, though might not be advisable from a public health perspective.

The forearm does not usually add much information for women who have had a hip and spine measurement. At this time, the total body bone mineral measurement is used mostly for research purposes and can also provide a very accurate assessment of body composition, including lean and fat mass. In some unusual circumstances, such as a condition called regional osteoporosis, the total body scan can be useful in following the resolution of the disease in a specific part of the body, distinct from the hip or spine.

The radiation exposure from central DXA readings is extremely low, about two to four mREMs. This is the equivalent of about one-twentieth of a standard chest X ray, one of the lowest-radiation procedures done, or the amount of radiation you would be exposed to while flying in an airplane from New York to Denver. Therefore, this should not be a consideration when determining if a bone density should be done, and/or what type should be done. Certainly, though, I would not advise anyone to have bone density measured while pregnant.

The bone mineral that is calculated by the scanner in a certain bone is divided by the area of the bone. A "true bone density" would actually require a correction for bone volume. Our current DXA scanners can only calculate two size dimensions at a time (height and width), so we correct the bone mineral content measured by the scanner by bone area instead of volume. This may not be as perfect as a true bone density corrected by bone volume, particularly in people who have very small or very large bones. For example, people who are very petite have a very small third dimension (depth of bone), whereas large people will have a very large third dimension. Therefore, if the very large person and the very small person both have the same measured BMD, it is likely to be an overestimate of true BMD in the very large person and an underestimate of true BMD in the very small person. Often I see petite women in the range of five feet or so who have very low BMD. I can reassure these women that their BMD is probably more normal for their small body size and bone size.

Overall, BMD is a great predictor of the risk of fracture. A one standard deviation (see below) reduction in bone density increases the risk of fracture by two to three times.

PERIPHERAL DXA AND SXA (SINGLE X-RAY ABSORPTIOMETRY)

Another way to measure bone density uses a similar technology, but measures peripheral bones and can be done in the heel or forearm (for example, the Lunar PIXI device) or finger (Schick accuDEXA device). When you look at large populations of people, all these tests can predict the risk of fractures. In other words, people who have a lower bone mass by any of these techniques are more likely to have fractures. When you look at hip fracture specifically, however, these tests are not quite as good as the hip DXA test at predicting the risk. Since the hip fracture is such an important fracture (from a personal as well as a public health and economic perspective), the hip BMD test is still preferable to these peripheral measures. When it comes to younger individuals—say, people between the ages of fifty and sixty—the lack of specific predictive value for hip fracture may not be so important, since hip fractures are quite rare in this age group. However, spine BMD, usually done with hip BMD, may have some advantages in this younger age group, since bone loss may be most marked in the spine in the first five to ten years after menopause. Therefore, spine BMD may be a bit more sensitive than peripheral DXA for picking up people at risk of osteoporotic fracture in the more recently postmenopausal group. There isn't much evidence to support this concept, however, since studies comparing different bone density techniques as they relate to vertebral fractures are few and far between.

There are some advantages to these peripheral measuring devices. Cost is one. Because the machines are small, they do not require a large office or room to accommodate them, so the rent space is cheaper. Furthermore, the capital cost to purchase the machines is lower than for the central dual X-ray machines. Therefore, the Medicare-approved charge for this measurement is about one-third to one-half of the approved charge for central DXA. The peripheral devices are more easily portable than the central machines because they are so small, so they are more likely to be used at health fairs and in private doctors' offices.

They are also incredibly fast: Bone mass measurements can be completed within one or two minutes. If you have a peripheral DXA or SXA measurement that is borderline or low, you may want to confirm the result with a central DXA test.

ULTRASOUND

A completely distinct way to measure bone mass uses ultrasound rather than X ray as the basis for the measurement. It produces a result in both speed of sound, as it moves through the bone and overlying soft tissue, as well as in broadband attenuation, or how much of the sound wave is lost as it travels through the part of the body being measured. This technique exposes a person to no radiation since it uses sound rather than X ray, and does not require a radiologic technologist to do the measurement. The machine is easily portable and has the other advantages stated above for other peripheral machines. It usually measures bone in the heel, but can also measure the forearm and tibia. It lacks the extremely high predictive value for hip fracture as the hip DXA has, but is highly predictive of all fractures.

One of the features that distinguishes this technique (ultrasound) from the techniques above (DXA and SXA) is its lower precision. *Precision* refers to the error involved in repeat measurements (even when there is no true change in bone mass). In other words, if a bone density test is repeated ten times in one morning, obviously bone density is not changing so fast; however, the measurements of bone density will differ slightly. The percent difference is calculated as the precision error or reliability of the technique. This is true of all biological measurements. For example, blood pressure measurement differs slightly minute by minute. Cholesterol measurements vary up and down, with or without modification of diet or addition of medication. The precision of ultrasound is slightly lower than the precision of DXA and SXA. Therefore it might not be as good for the monitoring of treatment or change in bone mass, where the best precision is needed to determine if small changes are occurring. If you have an equivocal or low measurement, you may want to confirm results with a central DXA test.

QUANTITATIVE COMPUTED TOMOGRAPHY (QCT)

Most CT scanners are able to also measure bone density of the spine, although the majority of these devices cannot currently measure bone density in other areas. There is an advantage of QCT in some instances: It can measure the spine BMD in the vertebral body, where fractures usually occur, and avoid the extra elements behind the body of the vertebrae where arthritis artifact usually affects measurement. This may be important for those people in whom degenerative disease prevents accurate spine BMD assessment by DXA and where the spine measurement is specifically needed, in addition to the hip measurement. In general, though, because this technique has poorer precision than the other techniques, and involves a substantially higher radiation exposure, it is not recommended for most patients as a bone density screening tool.

HAND RADIOGRAPHS

An X-ray-based technique in which the hands are measured alongside an aluminum wedge can also be used to measure density. Results are sent to a central processing center for computer determination of bone density. Although this technique can be portable, it does require central processing, so results may not be available as soon as they are for the techniques (above) in which the bone density is calculated on site immediately after the measurement is performed.

REPORTING BONE MASS

This part of the chapter discusses the way bone density results are reported, as well as explaining T- and Z-Scores and how osteoporosis and osteopenia are defined by T-Scores. I will also touch on differences in bone density related to gender and race.

Results from hip and spine DXA measurements are actually first calculated as grams of mineral per area of bone. Each bone normally has a different bone density. In order to standardize results across different sites and technologies, bone density measures are usually reported as T-Scores and Z-Scores. These have caused much confusion among doctors, as well as patients.

What Is a T-Score?

T-Scores are calculated from an individual's bone density results, the variation in bone density measurement, and the average bone density of a young normal reference population at peak bone mass. The age of the young normal reference population used to determine T-Scores differs slightly among different manufacturers of bone density measurement devices, but is usually between twenty and thirty-five years. This is the age when bone density is at its peak and osteoporosis-related fracture risk is at its lowest. Results are expressed as standard deviation (SD) scores above or below the average measurement for the young normal. A T-Score of –2 indicates that the person's score is 2 standard deviations below average for a young normal person of the same gender. On average, every T-Score above or below 0 represents about 10 to 15 percent reduction (or increment) in bone mass. For example, a T-Score of –2 in the spine means that the person's bone mass is about 20 percent lower in the spine than the average for a young normal person of the same gender.

Osteoporosis is defined by the T-Score, as originally decided by the World Health Organization (WHO) in 1992. A T-Score of –2.5 or lower indicates the presence of osteoporosis. An intermediate condition, called osteopenia or low bone mass, is defined as a T-Score between –1 and –2.5. The WHO criteria were designed as descriptive terms in order to determine the prevalence of bone mass at different levels in different populations. These cut points were never intended as treatment or diagnostic cut points. It turns out that the osteoporosis cut point actually makes some biologic sense; the risk of fracture is substantially increased at –2.5, and the majority of people do not reach this level until they are in their eighties. Furthermore, –2.5 seems to be the T-score at which treatment, at least with bisphosphonates, consistently works (see chapter 17). For example, in the alendronate clinical trials, alendronate reduced the risk of hip fractures in women who had T-Scores of –2.5 or lower but not in women with higher T-Scores. Similarly, in the risedronate clinical trial, risedronate only worked against hip fracture in those women who had documented osteoporosis. In contrast to *osteoporosis,* though, *osteopenia* does not make much sense as a diagnostic or therapeutic term.

What Is a Z-Score?

It is useful to know how your bone density compares with others of your age, even though that is not the way we define osteoporosis. The Z-Score compares a person's results to those of an average reference population of the same age and gender (as opposed to the T-Score, which compares the patient's measurement to that of a young population at peak bone mass). Just as for the T-Score, the Z-Score also takes into account the variability in the normal age-matched population. The results are expressed as positive or negative scores, referring to measurements above or below the average for the reference population. A score between −2 and +2 includes 95 percent of the population. Therefore, if you have a −2, you are in the lower 5th percentile for your age. If you have a Z-Score of +2, you are in the highest 95th percentile for your age. A score of 0 means that the person's bone density is exactly average for age and gender. A score of −1 means that that individual has a bone density one standard deviation below the average. For the spine, this usually means the BMD level is about 10 percent below the average. A score of −2 means that that individual's bone density is two SDs below the average, usually about 20 percent lower than the average spine BMD. In the hip region, the variability is a bit higher, so a score of −1 usually indicates a reduction of about 13 percent compared to the average, or 26 percent compared to the average when the Z-Score is reported as −2.

For every reduction in Z-Score, the risk of fracture increases approximately twofold. That is, if the person's Z-Score is −1, her risk of fracture is twice that of the average person at her age; for a score of −2, the person's risk of fracture is four times higher than the average person's; for a score of −3, the person's risk of fracture is eight times higher than the average. These differences are called relative risk; we ascertain one person's risk compared to the average person's. This still does not tell you how likely you are overall to have a fracture, however. That is called the absolute risk (see below).

Because almost everyone loses some bone with increasing age, it is difficult to avoid falling into the osteoporosis category if you live long enough. While only 13 percent of women be-

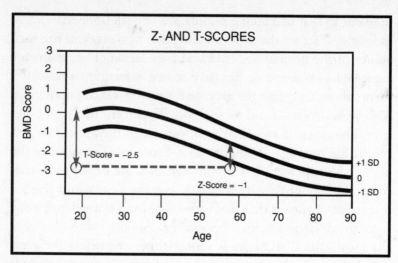

Figure 10-1: Each point reduction in a Z-score means twice the risk of fracture.

tween ages fifty and fifty-nine have osteoporosis, 27 percent of those between sixty and sixty-nine have osteoporosis, 47 percent of women between the ages of seventy and seventy-nine have osteoporosis, and 67 percent between eighty and eight-nine have osteoporosis.

OSTEOPENIA

Many people are distressed to learn that they have osteopenia. Since the term *osteopenia* implies that bone mass is slightly low but very much within normal limits, it should not be cause for alarm. Let's set the record straight: Osteopenia is not an affliction or a disease. In fact, almost no woman can escape a label of osteopenia if she lives long enough. For example, although 60 percent of people in their fifties have BMD above the osteopenic range, 40 percent have BMD levels in the osteopenic range or below. Among those in their sixties, the majority of women have bone density values in the osteopenic range or below; only 40 percent have normal BMD levels. When women reach their seventies, less than 20 percent have normal

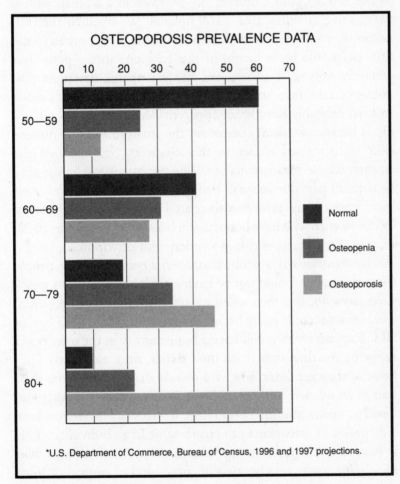

Figure 10-2: The majority of women over the age of sixty have bone density in either the osteopenic or osteoporotic range.

BMD levels, and in their eighties, it's only 10 percent who have BMD measurements above the osteopenic levels.

Osteopenia means that your bone density could fall anywhere between the lower fifth to sixteenth percentile compared to the average young normal BMD. Even in a woman who is twenty-five or thirty, this is still normal. We consider the fifth percentile to be normal with respect to height. A woman in the fifth percentile has a height of five feet, one inch—petite but certainly normal. Furthermore, the osteopenia determination does not take into account body size. We know that smaller women probably have lower apparent BMD the way we measure it because we don't correct for the small third bone dimension (as discussed earlier in this chapter). So, many of the women whose measurements fall in the osteopenic range may be there in part due to small body size and small bone size. And most importantly, osteoporosis-related fracture risk is extremely low in women who have bone mass in this range (see figure 10-3), in contrast to fracture risk in women with osteoporosis.

So *osteopenia* is a problematic term even in young people (who in general should not be having their bone densities measured anyway). But then when we start "diagnosing osteopenia" in older women, it really becomes ludicrous. More than half of all Caucasian women will have a bone density in the osteopenia range by the time they reach their sixties, since everybody loses bone as they get older. To give a disease diagnosis to more than half of all women in their middle age, when they are otherwise healthy, makes absolutely no sense. Moreover, I have seen how a diagnosis of osteopenia can create panic in an individual. This is particularly true in young women. I have had patients who have gone to doctors because of some kind of muscle or joint pain and somehow ended up getting a bone density test. In one of the most egregious cases, a young woman aged thirty had a

Undiagnosed Low BMD in Postmenopausal Women

	Fracture Rate (SE)		
Fracture Type	**T>−1.0 (Normal)**	**−1.0>T>−2.5 (Osteopenic)**	**T≤−2.5 (Osteoporotic)**
Any osteoporotic fracture	0.86 (0.024)	1.55 (0.044)	3.47 (0.160)
Hip	0.10 (0.009)	0.27 (0.019)	0.89 (0.082)
Spine	0.09 (0.009)	0.17 (0.014)	0.45 (0.058)
Rib	0.23 (0.014)	0.43 (0.023)	0.88 (0.081)
Wrist	0.22 (0.014)	0.61 (0.023)	1.17 (0.094)
Forearm	0.09 (0.009)	0.14 (0.013)	0.26 (0.044)

Figure 10-3: Fracture rates per 100 person-years of follow-up according to T-Score.

BMD measurement showing her to be in the osteopenic range. In her follow-up consultation with her doctor, she was told that she might end up in a nursing home in a few years. She was specifically told to curtail all outdoor recreational and sporting activities and to be very careful walking down stairs. While the latter comment might be good general advice, the other comments are completely outrageous. Fracture risk is very low in a woman with low bone density alone, and life is very short. The advantages of living an active lifestyle far outweigh the disadvantages, for the health of both bone and other organ systems. Furthermore, this woman was told to start a medication because of her severe condition, which has not been tested at all in healthy young women. Who knows what it would do in a woman of childbearing age? It is often difficult to justify starting medication even in an older woman with osteopenia who has age as a risk factor, but it is almost impossible to justify starting medication in a younger woman with osteopenia (assuming no other major manifestations of osteoporosis).

To get a better sense of how low your bone mass is, it is much more reasonable to consider your bone mass compared to your peers (your Z-Score). Even more important, though, is to understand the likelihood of having an osteoporosis-related fracture by considering your absolute risk of fracturing.

FACTORS BESIDES AGE THAT INFLUENCE BONE DENSITY: GENDER AND RACE

Most of the information that we have about osteoporosis, bone density, and fracture risk is based on Caucasian women since osteoporosis is so much more common in this group. African American women have higher bone mass values than Caucasian women, and African American men have higher bone mass values than white men. African Americans of both genders have a lower fracture risk than their Caucasian counterparts. Likewise, men overall have less fracture risk than women.

We are still gathering information about groups other than white women. The current standard for bone density reporting is to define osteoporosis in men and non-Caucasians in a way similar to that done in white women. Z- and T-Scores are usually reported according to the reference populations specific for that age and gender. Doing it this way, the risk of fracture in men with a T-Score based on normal male populations is similar to that in women with that same T-Score. Since treatment guidelines need to be based on absolute fracture risk, this approach is reasonable and what most bone density machine outputs currently do. Similar arguments might apply to women of other ethnicities, though this is still being worked out.

DISCREPANCIES BETWEEN ONE SKELETAL SITE AND ANOTHER

Some people have a low bone mass in one bone and a normal bone mass in another. As discussed previously, this may be related to scoliosis, arthritis, fractures, or calcifications overlying the spine in the case where the spinal bone mass is much higher than the hip, particularly in older individuals. However, there may also be a genetic pattern in which an individual seems to inherit a tendency to have low bone mass at one site versus another. Why this might occur is not known. It could relate to hormonal factors, mechanical factors, variability in bone size, and more. It can also occur in the reverse: People sometimes have normal hip values and very low spine values. Again, genetics may account for this. It is logical to assume in a case like this that the person will have a high risk for spinal fracture and a lower or intermediate risk for fracture at nonvertebral regions. This has not been proven, in part because this is not the common situation. Medications can also produce a discrepancy between one site and another. Steroid drugs, for example, can reduce bone mass in the spine more than in the hip and produce osteoporosis in one site rather than another. In my opinion, it is clinically reasonable to make treatment recommendations based on the lowest bone density measurement.

THE BARE BONES

- If you are at risk of osteoporosis, you must get a bone density test when you reach the appropriate stage in life.
- If you have access to a central dual X-ray absorptiometry test, this is the preferred method of assessment.

- If you do not have ready access to the central DXA test, you should get a bone density using whatever technique is available.
- The interpretation of the bone density measurement and the determination about whether treatment is indicated may be far more important than the decision about which bone density test to have.
- If you have a peripheral measurement of any type and the results are equivocal about your risk of osteoporosis, you should proceed, if possible, with a measurement of hip and spine by central DXA to confirm the diagnosis.
- Bone density tests usually report your results in comparison to the average of healthy individuals of your same age and gender (Z-Score) as well as to the average of healthy young normal individuals (T-Score).
- In order to figure out how much worse your bone density is compared to other women of your age, you need to know your Z-Score.
- In the future, the reporting of T- and Z-Scores for bone density will probably change. We will move toward reporting of absolute risk of fracture based on bone density level as well as age and other risk factors such as having had a prior fracture.
- If you get a bone density and the results show osteopenia, don't panic. This may be normal for your age. Still, you should talk to your doctor about it; if you are postmenopausal and have certain risk factors, you may be in a category where medical treatment is recommended.

Chapter 11

Blood and Urine Tests and
Radiologic Procedures

Among patients who have very low bone mass—particularly if the bone mass is low for the person's age (a Z-Score of –2 or less)—it might sometimes be reasonable to obtain certain blood and urine tests. These are useful to determine if any underlying, previously unrecognized disease might be contributing to the osteoporosis. There are not particularly clear guidelines here, and your doctor will have to use her or his judgment to determine what makes sense for you depending on your prior medical history, any ongoing symptoms you might have, how low your bone mass is, and whether you have had any fractures. This chapter briefly describes the possible blood and urine tests that might be done, the other radiology procedures that might be requested, and the rarely used bone biopsy.

Some of the tests that should be considered are routine blood tests often done for other purposes anyway, including complete blood counts, kidney function tests, liver function tests, calcium level and thyroid function tests (especially the pituitary hormone TSH, to exclude overactivity of the thyroid gland).

Many of the more specialized tests are discussed below. It would be completely unnecessary for these tests to be done in the vast majority of patients. So unless you are a woman who has already been found to have a very low BMD measurement for your age, you can skip this chapter. If you are one of these women, or if you have not responded as well to osteoporosis treatment as your doctor feels you should have, then some of the following tests might be reasonable for your doctor to consider. It's useful to have an idea what some of these tests are so you can specifically question your physician.

SPECIALIZED TESTS TO EXCLUDE UNDERLYING DISEASES

• **Parathyroid hormone level to exclude primary hyperparathyroidism.** Parathyroid hormone is completely unrelated to thyroid hormone. Its name derives from the proximity of the parathyroid gland to the thyroid gland in the front of the lower neck. It is the hormone largely responsible for maintaining normal levels of calcium in the blood. Excessive levels may be a result of a tumor (almost always benign). This condition, called hyperparathyroidism, can result in excessive loss of bone and elevated levels of calcium in the blood. In many cases, a minor surgical procedure may be required to remove the benign tumor.

• **Vitamin D level to exclude deficiency or insufficiency.** It is still not clear what the level of vitamin D should be for optimal bone health, and in general we recommend supplementation with 400 to 800 IU of vitamin D per day depending on age without measuring this level (as discussed in chapter 6).

Sometimes, however, in patients with very low bone mass, it might make sense to measure the blood level to make sure that more vitamin D is not needed.

• **Protein subclasses in the blood to identify a blood disease called multiple myeloma** (a test called protein electrophoresis). Usually, abnormalities on this test are from benign conditions, but in some circumstances evaluation by a hematologist and further testing may be required. If this test is seriously abnormal, there will often be other signs or symptoms of the disease, but on rare occasions osteoporosis may be the only manifestation.

• **Transglutaminase antibodies to exclude a malabsorption disease called celiac disease.** Another name for this disease is gluten-sensitive enteropathy. It changes the shape of the intestinal lining such that it cannot absorb some of the nutrients that pass by it, including calcium and vitamin D. It often causes abdominal discomfort, diarrhea, and excessive gas, but sometimes the symptoms may be subtle or even nonexistent. It is usually treated effectively with a diet that strictly avoids gluten products and provides adequate calcium and vitamin D including supplements when needed. This is a difficult diet to follow, so a definitive diagnosis must be made before it should be undertaken. The definitive diagnosis may require an upper endoscopy with biopsy of the small intestine.

• **Cortisol levels in a twenty-four-hour urine collection or blood cortisol levels after suppression with dexamethasone to look for Cushing's syndrome.** Use of steroids or glucocorticoids for the treatment of certain medical conditions is well known to produce adverse effects on the skeleton. There are also diseases in which the body itself overproduces these chemicals. This endogenous hyperproduction can produce the same problems for bones as the medical treatment does. One of the common pathologic conditions that produces excess steroids in the body is a pituitary tumor (almost always benign). A CT or MRI of the brain is required if this diagnosis is being considered, but more intensive testing might also be necessary. Referral to an endocrinologist is also mandatory. While this disease may have other symptoms or signs associated with it, it does sometimes present in this subtle way with osteoporosis as the only manifestation.

• **Urine calcium levels to exclude excessive calcium excretion.** Sometimes people experience an obligatory excretion of calcium in the urine that exceeds the normal. Without efforts to modify this excretion and supplement calcium in the diet to make up for this daily deficit, it might produce a drain on the skeleton. The body dissolves bone in order to keep the blood calcium levels normal while calcium is pouring out through the kidney. Furthermore, high urine calcium concentrations might increase the risk of kidney stones. Certainly anyone with a history of kidney stones and osteoporosis should have the twenty-four-hour collection analyzed for calcium. If excessive calcium excretion is found, it can be treated, sometimes effectively, with a thiazide-containing diuretic (water pill). Thiazides cause more calcium to be reabsorbed back from the kidney tubules into the blood, reducing the magnitude of urinary calcium losses.

• In rare circumstances, when patients have flushing, hives, allergies, skin rashes, or diarrhea, a diagnosis of mastocytosis should be considered. Blood levels of an enzyme called tryptase may be useful and referral to a hematologist may be required.

TESTS OF BONE TURNOVER

Sometimes tests of either the urine or blood can be useful in determining the degree of bone turnover in an individual patient. These are biochemical tests that indicate how fast the bone is remodeling. Bone turnover levels reflect the dynamic status of the skeleton—how quickly or actively bone is remodeling at the moment. An elevation in bone turnover may be a clue to the fact that bone quality is suboptimal. For example, elevated turnover may cause microscopic structural damage within the bone or prevent the bone from achieving the normal amount of bone mineral. It may be associated with the development of holes in the outer margins of the bone. Therefore, these tests can be useful to help in predicting a person's individual risk of fracturing. Even more importantly, they may be helpful in determining whether a treatment is actually working for osteoporosis.

Levels of bone remodeling or bone turnover are increased at the time of menopause and with advancing age in most individuals. Being immobilized can affect bone turnover. Certain diseases can also elevate bone turnover, such as rheumatoid arthritis.

The information these tests provide is totally distinct from the information provided by bone density testing. Bone density changes slowly (over years), whereas bone turnover can vary over weeks to months. Bone density represents a result of all of the good and bad things that have happened to the skeleton over the entire lifetime of an individual. In contrast, bone turnover represents only what is happening that day and not previously. Thus bone turnover tests could never take the place of bone density testing for the diagnosis of osteoporosis. They can supply additional information, however, that bone density cannot provide.

There are a number of different bone turnover tests, and we do not have sufficient data from comparative studies to determine if one test has an obvious advantage over another. They include blood tests that measure rates of bone formation called osteocalcin and bone-specific alkaline phosphatase, and propeptides of procollagen as well as blood or urine tests called n-telopeptide (NTX) or c-telopeptide (CTX) and urine tests for pyridinium crosslinks (DPD or PYD), all of which measure levels of bone resorption.

Measuring these levels is not necessary in everyone. There are, however, some clinical situations in which measuring the levels might be useful. If risk factors and bone density level are borderline and it is not clear whether a patient should be treated with osteoporosis medication, a marker of bone turnover might help sway the decision. If the marker is high, it may be considered an independent risk factor for fracturing. Therefore, if the other measurements do not mandate therapy, the addition of a high bone turnover level may mandate therapy.

Bone turnover marker levels can also be used to help determine whether medical treatments are working. Levels that are substantially reduced after treatment may help reassure patient and doctor that the treatment is having the desired effect. This may be particularly important in a condition that is largely asymptomatic in its early stages. Unfortunately, these tests normally feature a lot of hour-to-hour and day-to-day variability, so big changes are required to be sure that a difference in level is really related to the medication rather than just test variability. It is sometimes necessary to repeat the marker level determination in order to interpret the test correctly.

Also, when obtaining these tests, it is ideal to have each sample obtained at approximately the same time of day. There is a diurnal rhythm to the levels of these substances in the blood and urine—that is, the average levels change over the course of the day and night. To get the most accurate assessment of change in level, then, the second level should be obtained at the same time as the first. There are also some tests that vary substantially with food consumption, such that the ideal time to measure these levels is in the morning before breakfast. For the urine tests, we usually recommend the second morning fasting sample of urine. This means that the first urine of the morning should be discarded, but the next time a person can urinate—usually within about two hours—prior to eating breakfast, a small sample of urine should be collected and then brought to the clinical laboratory.

Bone marker tests may also be useful for monitoring patients who are being treated with medication and have been changed to a new bone density machine for the follow-up measurement. Follow-up bone density tests are best done on the same machine as the first measurement. When this is impossible, it limits the conclusions we can draw about bone mass stability, gain, or loss. In this circumstance, the marker can help determine the dynamic status of bone, and help confirm that treatment is working.

X RAYS

Obviously, any possible fracture must be diagnosed with an X ray of the injured area. Usually, specific treatment is required to help the fracture heal (splinting, casting, or sometimes surgical fixation of the broken bones). Rib fractures, however, are often not specifically treated; they heal spontaneously with no intervention.

For the spine, sometimes X rays should be obtained even without specific episodes of back pain. As discussed in an earlier chapter, vertebral compressions (fractures) from osteoporosis sometimes occur with no clear pain syndrome. Sometimes the evidence that a person might have a compression fracture is a history of loss of height (usually more than one to one and a half inches), or a change in the shape of the back or torso (frequently forward stooping or the classic dowager's hump). Any person who has osteoporosis or bone mass close to the osteoporosis range and experiences back pain, substantial height loss, or postural change should have a lateral X ray of the thoracic and lumbar spine. It is important to note that many people who have had low back pain have had lumbar X rays, but often thoracic (between the neck and the lower back) spine X rays are not done in this context.

The reason that back X rays are so strongly recommended is that even a compression found on X ray that is completely unassociated with symptoms increases the risk of further fractures quite dramatically; eventually these fractures can produce symptoms, particularly if more than one compression fracture occurs. These symptoms can occur years later and include back pain, height loss, postural change, restricted breathing, and abdominal symptoms. It is therefore extremely important that these abnormalities be found. Anyone who has one should be treated with anti-osteoporosis medication, in addition to appropriate modification of nutrition and exercise.

In the process of doing clinical research studies in osteoporosis, we often have patients with borderline bone densities who go for X rays as part of the screening process to see if they can participate. Many times, the X ray will reveal a bone deformity or compression that would never have otherwise been found. Also common are stories of women who have experienced some change in the shape of their backs as well as some height loss; these women not uncommonly are found to have several vertebral compressions on X ray. The use of a new tool called instant morphometric, or lateral vertebral imaging, that's available on state-of-the-art bone density testing machines, may allow us to diagnose many of these deformities without sending the patient for another test. This will be a wonderful way to identify more women and men who need treatment for osteoporosis, since ultimately many will get into trouble as a result of these initially asymptomatic fractures.

BONE SCANS AND MRI

Much back pain is unrelated to osteoporosis. Among the most common causes are arthritis, degenerative disk disease (herniated or bulging disks), muscle strain, and ligament sprain. Sometimes additional imaging tests besides the plain X ray are used to help diagnose these conditions. These tests are not usually required to diagnose osteoporosis. It is important to realize that these conditions can all coexist. It used to be thought that people with arthritis of the spine were less likely to have osteoporosis of the spine. In part, this concept was related to the fact that obesity increases the risk of arthritis, while it decreases the risk of osteoporosis. In fact, both of these diseases are very common and increase in prevalence with increasing age; by no means should a diagnosis of one exclude a diagnosis of the other. Furthermore, one of the complications of vertebral compression fractures might be arthritic deterioration as a result of abnormal forces crossing the bone and joint spaces.

In a person who has cancer, doctors sometimes may recommend a bone scan in which a minute amount of radioactive material is injected into a vein to see if the cancer has spread. This type of test can also be used to diagnose a bone infection or confirm a fracture. Vertebral compressions can appear similarly to cancer or infections on this test. This type of bone scan is completely distinct from a bone density test (BMD), though the BMD tests are sometimes also called bone scans. As stated earlier, bone density (BMD) tests do not require an intravenous line or any contrast material. In contrast to the bone scan, the bone density test is completely noninvasive and takes only about ten minutes, compared to hours required to complete the bone scan.

MRI tests are also not usually needed for osteoporosis-related complications. These tests are particularly useful to distinguish osteoporosis-related abnormalities from cancer-related abnormalities and other degenerative processes involving nerves and joint spaces.

BONE BIOPSY OF THE ILIAC CREST

This is a procedure performed under a local anesthetic, often in a treatment or procedure room rather than a true operating room. A small core of bone is removed from the iliac crest— the large bone that shapes your hips and that you can easily feel beginning just below your waist. The procedure is performed under a local anesthetic, sometimes accompanied by a relaxing agent given through a vein. With modern techniques, there is usually little discomfort while the procedure is being performed. Since the iliac crest is a non-weight-bearing bone, there is absolutely no danger in removing a small piece of it.

Transiliac bone biopsies are performed electively after taking tetracycline antibiotics for a few days several weeks prior to the procedure. Tetracycline antibiotics actually are incorporated into remodeling bone as it is becoming mineralized and can allow calculation of the rate of bone remodeling, specifically bone mineralization. For this purpose, the bone biopsy has been largely supplanted by tests of bone turnover (see above) in the blood or urine. The major use of the bone biopsy now is for research purposes. Extracting a small piece of bone allows us to calculate the amount of bone mineral, the microscopic architecture of bone, and the concentration and health of bone cells. Assessing these allows us to help determine the mechanisms of action of medications effective in treating osteoporosis. However, the transiliac crest bone biopsy might be useful on a rare occasion for clinical purposes to exclude some rare causes of osteoporosis, such as mastocytosis, an excess of a type of immune cell. This can produce bone dissolution as well as diarrhea, flushing, and rashes among other symptoms.

THE BARE BONES

- In most cases, osteoporosis is diagnosed by bone density testing alone; blood and urine tests are not required.
- Blood and urine tests for bone turnover, such as n-telopeptide or NTX, can be adjunctive to bone density tests in predicting risk of fractures and in determining if osteoporosis treatment is working.
- If bone turnover markers are to be utilized for treatment monitoring, levels should be obtained before initiating therapy and compared to those obtained four to six months after treatment.
- In patients with back pain, height loss of one or more inches, or changes in posture, X rays of the spine (middle

and lower) should be performed to determine if there are any compression fractures. Certain bone density testing equipment can also diagnose these abnormalities.

- Other imaging tests called radionuclide bone scans or MRI tests are needed only rarely, usually to exclude other non-osteoporosis causes of back pain.

- Specialized blood and urine tests may be recommended if your bone density is very low compared to age-matched peers, if you have multiple fractures, if you are losing bone rapidly, or if your treatment appears to be ineffective.

- The special tests that might be done will exclude diseases such as hyperthyroidism, hyperparathyroidism, vitamin D deficiency, multiple myeloma, celiac disease, Cushing's syndrome, mastocytosis, and excessive urine calcium excretion.

Part IV

MEDICATION
AND
TREATMENT

Chapter 12

Fracture Care and Rehabilitation

This chapter focuses primarily on the medical treatment of vertebral or spine fractures—including medication, physical therapy, and bracing—and also overviews relatively recent procedures for persistently painful vertebral fractures called vertebroplasty and kyphoplasty. As stated earlier, the majority of back pain is not due to osteoporosis. The only way to determine whether back pain might be a consequence of osteoporosis is to perform an X ray of the spine (and/or obtain a lateral view of the spine on a DXA device). This chapter assumes that the diagnosis of fracture has already been made; it is my hope that this information will help patients live well with osteoporosis, reduce symptoms of chronic pain, and help prevent further fractures from occurring. The chapter also touches on general approaches to management of other fractures, usually handled by orthopedists.

Since fractures and their consequences are the only outcomes we really care about in osteoporosis treatment, it is important to make brief mention of how we treat them. The treatment of osteoporosis-related fractures is largely the domain of the orthopedist. I am not an orthopedist, so I will not provide any details about fracture repair. As an endocrinologist and osteoporosis specialist, my mission is to use any medical or other means to prevent the first fracture by identifying and treating the person at risk, as well as to reduce the risk of subsequent fractures in people who have already had them. This involves recognizing, diagnosing, and treating the underlying disease. Some orthopedists treat the fracture but do not look further for the underlying cause of the fracture or consider the possibility of using medical therapy to reduce the risk of future fractures.

Usually fractures result in emergency room visits, with X rays and orthopedic consultation. On occasion, with less severe fractures or fractures of smaller bones (fingers or toes), people avoid the emergency room and wait until they can make a direct visit to an orthopedist's office. When people sustain hip fractures, an immediate or urgent surgery is almost always required. There are three types of surgeries that are often performed. One is a nail, pin, and/or screw fixation. Another, a partial hip replacement, is used for fractures in which there is sufficient damage to the blood supply to predict that the fracture won't heal. A total hip replacement is generally done when significant arthritis accompanies the fracture. These are orthopedic decisions based on the location and severity of the fracture, the presence and degree of displacement of the two broken ends of bone, and the health of the joint space.

Many distal leg fractures (of the thigh- or shinbone) also require surgical repair, though sometimes casting is appropriate. A common osteoporosis-related fracture is of the shoulder or proximal humerus. This fracture can often be treated with sling immobilization although surgical fixation or sometimes even shoulder replacement might be required. Wrist or forearm fractures are usually handled with external reduction (manually putting the pieces back together) and casting.

Certain fractures do not require orthopedic consultation because no specific reduction or immobilization is required. These include rib and vertebral fractures. Most osteoporosis-related rib fractures produce substantial pain but do not result in any complications and heal spontaneously. In contrast, rib fractures due to serious trauma may be associated with a piece of bone puncturing lung tissue and require emergency treatment. Most osteoporosis-related rib fractures are simply handled with pain medicine and reduced activity as needed until the pain improves.

THE TREATMENT OF PAINFUL VERTEBRAL FRACTURES

I have had patients who go the emergency room of the nearby hospital with vertebral fractures and subsequently require hospitalization to control their pain. Some of these individuals don't recover quickly enough and are transferred to an inpatient rehabilitation program. Often, my patients who have suffered acute vertebral fractures have stated that it is the worst pain they have ever felt, including childbirth. In addition to the bone pain, women sometimes suffer from intense back muscle spasms that can accompany the fracture. These create pain so severe, it can take your breath away.

Most patients can be treated as outpatients, however. The treatment of acute vertebral fractures is primarily medical (though often treatment is administered by an orthopedist). The major initial goal is to relieve the pain; there is no need to fix the fracture. Pain medication can be over-the-counter agents such as acetaminophen, anti-inflammatory pain medicines such as ibuprofen, or the newer but related class of prescription medicines called COX-2 inhibitors (Celebrex or Vioxx or Bextra), which are longer lasting and are less irritating to the stomach. These may be insufficient in some individuals, and narcotic pain medicines may be required (oxycodone, codeine). Moist or dry heating pads can offer some relief, as does sitting or floating in hot therapeutic pools. Muscle spasm might require treatment with a muscle relaxant. Constipation often accompanies acute vertebral fractures and should be treated with bowel softeners and/or cathartics.

Temporary reduction in activity is usually required, but activity should be continued as much as tolerated. It is particularly important for people with osteoporosis not to be relegated to long periods of bed rest, which will only exacerbate bone loss and make future fractures more likely. There are no hard-and-fast rules here. Vertebral compression is very different from a long-bone fracture. There is no need to immobilize the ends of the bone. Many people think that the compressed or fractured bone is actually more stable than the original unaffected bone. Therefore, there is no clear period of time during which activity must cease. The period of rest is normally determined by how much pain the individual is in, and how activity affects the pain. Each patient must make her or his own individual judgment. In general, light activity—at least a bit of walking in the house—is preferable to bed rest, since bed rest is detrimental to the underlying bone.

Outpatient physical therapy may be helpful to teach people who have experienced vertebral fractures to avoid certain movements, such as forward bending of the spine and rotation or twisting of the torso. Heavy lifting should be avoided; even light lifting must be done with particular attention to appropriate protective body mechanics. Other movements to avoid are those involving high impact on the vertebrae or exaggerated reaching, particularly when associated with forward movement. Physical therapy should also concentrate on exercising the postural or spinal muscles (see figures 7-1 and 7-2). These exercises include arching the back, doing modified push-ups against the wall, positioning yourself on hands and knees and performing leg extensions, and stretching with the arms bent to try to get the elbows to meet in the back (see chapter 7). Whenever a person can be conscious of it—hopefully multiple times during the day—an effort should be made to sit up very tall and straight, to elevate the head, and to keep the shoulders back and down. It is thought that these positions, movements, and exercises can help prevent further vertebral fractures; still, anyone who has had a fracture is at substantially higher risk of having another one. As a result, we know that all patients who have suffered a vertebral fracture should receive specific medical treatment for osteoporosis (see chapter 11). The risk of a second vertebral fracture seems particularly high in the first year following a vertebral fracture. These multiple vertebral fracture episodes seem to cluster in time.

Sometimes back braces are prescribed. One type is a stiff plastic-and-metal immobilizer meant to stabilize the fracture. There is really no evidence whatsoever that this bracing has any impact at all on the outcome of the fracture. In fact, neurologic problems related to movement of the fractured bone are extremely rare—almost unheard of with osteoporotic vertebral compressions. These braces are very uncomfortable. One of my first experiences as an osteoporosis specialist was with a patient who had experienced a recent vertebral compression. In a large shopping bag, she carried the brace that she had been given but could not wear. Since she had been told to wear the brace anytime she was out of bed, she simply stayed in bed. Finally, she correctly realized that this could not be helping her situation. I've observed this phenomenon numerous times over the course of my career.

A second type of back brace that patients have told me can help reduce discomfort is a girdle-type elastic band that fastens with Velcro for proper fit. Many patients find this to give them a little extra security and comfort as they start moving again after the pain subsides. As with the stiff brace above, there is really no evidence base to support the use of this brace, but it is reasonable to try it in the early stages of pain. A posture-training support device that looks like a small backpack can help keep the spine erect and in proper alignment with the hips and help keep the shoulders back. Small weights can be added as tolerated. This device can help relieve back pain from vertebral fractures and help train correct posture. In the long run, though, it is best to avoid back support devices, which can contribute to weakening of the underlying muscles. These should be used for symptom relief for as short a period of time as possible.

After the initial pain is gone, a course of physical therapy including teaching of proper body mechanics—especially avoidance of spinal flexion—and a back extension exercise program may be beneficial to help prevent subsequent fractures. Again, most of these recommendations are based on clinical experience and not on good controlled research studies.

VERTEBROPLASTY/KYPHOPLASTY PROCEDURES

Pain from a vertebral fracture usually improves within a few days but may take two to six weeks to resolve completely. Rarely, patients have severe persistent pain beyond this period. Relatively new techniques called vertebroplasty and kyphoplasty may be performed in these individuals. Spine orthopedists, neurosurgeons, and invasive radiologists can all perform these procedures. There have been no randomized controlled trials to evaluate the effectiveness and safety of these procedures; all of our information so far is based on observation. These data suggest that the procedures are highly effective at relieving pain in those people suffering severe persistent pain from a relatively acute vertebral compression fracture (within a few months). Risks include cement leaking around the spinal cord, sometimes producing temporary paralysis and requiring surgical correction. Infection and risks associated with anesthesia used in any surgical procedure are also possible.

Usually, an MRI of the spine is performed to determine if there is still swelling within the affected bone and to select appropriate patients for the procedure. If all the swelling is gone, it may make it less likely that the procedure will help. Some of these procedures are done under a local anesthetic and some under a general. The basic technique is performed with the patient lying on her or his abdomen. Under X-ray guidance, a needle is inserted through the back into the affected bone of the spine. With vertebroplasty, cement is injected directly into the body of the crushed bone. With kyphoplasty, a small balloon is inflated once the needle is inserted into the appropriate place; then the cement or glue material is injected into the space created by the balloon. A full discussion of the relative benefits and risks of the two procedures is beyond the scope of this book, but anyone considering the procedures should talk them over thoroughly with her or his physician.

At this point, with limited available data, these procedures should be limited to use as a last resort for treatment of pain. The first referral I made for this procedure was about two years before this writing. The patient was an older woman who had had multiple vertebral fractures over about a year's time. Prior to this year, she had never had any knowledge about osteoporosis. She had already been to pain clinics and was on narcotic medication. Nevertheless she was extremely limited in her activity due to pain, and was persistently groggy from the medication. I decided to bite the bullet and refer her to an orthopedic colleague in New York City. She had the vertebroplasty procedure soon afterward. I spoke to her daughter the next day; she told me that her mom had experienced 90 percent pain relief as soon as she woke up from the procedure. Anecdotally, it is clear that the vertebroplasty and kyphoplasty techniques can be miraculous in relieving severe pain from a vertebral fracture.

Most people can recover from these fractures on their own, however. In the future, these procedures may become more standard for treatment of certain vertebral fractures even in the absence of severe pain. Kyphoplasty might have the potential to raise the height of the affected bone and return the shape of the bone to normal. Thus this procedure may be able to reverse the abnormal curvature sometimes seen with osteoporosis of the spine. This may improve the mechanics of the spine in the long run though there are no data confirming this. There is also some concern that by increasing the stiffness in the affected bone, the bone above or below might be subject to abnormal forces that could have a negative impact on the likelihood of fracture in these adjacent vertebrae. It is too early to tell at this point. A good randomized clinical trial is currently being planned to answer some of these questions. It is possible that at some point in the future we will look at this technique to stabilize a vertebral fracture the same way we now look at casting or nail and screw fixations of other fractures—but we are not there yet.

RECOGNIZING THE POSSIBILITY OF OSTEOPOROSIS

It is critical that anyone who suffers an adulthood fracture in the absence of a very traumatic accident (such as in a motor vehicle accident) recognize that osteoporosis may be a contributing factor. Many doctors who treat fractures as their primary profession do not discuss osteoporosis with their patients, yet the underlying disease must be recognized to prompt a bone density test, preventive measures, and medication when needed. Making this connection should be part of the acute treatment of fractures.

REHABILITATION PROGRAMS FOR PEOPLE WITH FRACTURES

It is clear that every effort should be made to avoid long periods of immobilization in patients with fractures. Immobilization results in rapid loss of bone and is likely to result in worsening osteoporosis risk. All patients who have had osteoporosis-related fractures are candidates for rehabilitation programs. Both inpatient and outpatient programs are available in many urban and suburban areas. Rehabilitation programs may be administered through rehabilitation doctors (physiatrists), medical doctors, and/or physical or occupational therapists.

Rehabilitation programs aim to keep people moving even during the early recovery from a serious fracture and provide advice about how to perform all the normal activities of daily living safely (getting out of bed and transferring to a chair or toilet, along with walking, bathing, grooming, cooking, and lifting) to avoid further injury or future falls. In a rehabilitation program, a person will be evaluated for the need to use assistive devices for walking (straight canes, four-legged canes, walkers with wheels, or walkers without wheels), as well as reaching, lifting, and grooming. In patients who have had back fractures, spine braces, corsets, or posture-training supports (which look like small backpacks) will be considered; hip pads or protectors might be recommended, particularly for people who are thin around the hip region and at high risk for hip fracture because of low bone density and/or frequent falls. All individuals will be given a therapeutic exercise program. The exercise regimen is aimed at trying to keep people active after fractures by using movements that do not harm and might actually help the recovery process. The ultimate goal of rehabilitation is to reduce pain, improve function, help a person maintain as much independence as possible, and improve quality of life. In some cases, these treatments can reduce the likelihood of future fractures.

SAFETY CONCEPTS FOR THE BACK

For people who are experiencing prolonged back pain after a vertebral fracture, short-term use of corsets, back braces, or posture-training supports may be suggested to reduce the load on the affected part of the back and maintain good spine alignment. In the long run, however, these devices might contribute to muscle weakening and therefore should only be continued if absolutely necessary.

There are several motions that are important to avoid in patients who have had prior vertebral fractures from osteoporosis. These are flexion or forward bending, and twisting or rotating the back. Both of these movements produce too much stress on the part of the vertebral bones that fracture in patients with osteoporosis and can precipitate worsening vertebral compression. Combining the two motions (forward bending and twisting) is particularly problematic. Extreme reaching, especially when reaching in front of the body, should be avoided, as should high impact activity or jumping on a hard surface (a trampoline with a handrail is probably okay).

Spine-Alignment Techniques

- When standing, walking, or sitting:
  - Keep your back straight.
  - Don't slump forward.
  - Keep your torso and chest lifted upright.
  - Keep your shoulders back.
  - Keep your head erect with eyes forward and chin up.
  - Gently tighten your abdominal muscles to keep the small of your back flat.
- When standing for a long time:
  - Keep one foot bent up on a stool, periodically switching this resting position to the other foot.
- When lifting:
  - Keep the object close to your body, bend at the hips and knees but not the abdomen, and keep your back straight.

- When tying shoes:
  - Put your foot on a stepstool so that you can comfortably bend at the waist to tie.
  - Avoid rounding your back.
- When sweeping or vacuuming:
  - Keep the broom or vacuum within comfortable range in front of you such that the movement can be done without bending your back forward.

SAFETY CONCEPTS: FALLS

The vast majority of osteoporosis-related fractures—including those of the hip and forearm as well as a substantial proportion of spine fractures—occur after falls. Therefore, the risk of fractures is dependent upon the strength of underlying bone as well as the likelihood of falling. Strategies to reduce falling risk are critical in the management of osteoporosis and prevention of future fractures.

To Reduce Falling Risk

- Evaluate home safety:
  - Make sure there are lights within reach of your bed.
  - Make sure the hallway between your bed and bathroom is sufficiently lit with a night-light, or use a flashlight to get to the bathroom during the night.

- Use rubber or adhesive strips in the bath-tub or shower.
- Wear shoes with low heels and nonslip soles.
- Don't wear excessively long clothing.
- Make sure handrails are available on both indoor and outdoor stairways.
- Be aware that certain medications can make you drowsy and make falling more likely.
- Avoid loose throw rugs and cluttered walk-ways.
- Be conscious of outdoor safety:
  - Avoid walking on slippery surfaces.
  - Look carefully for cracks and uneven road and sidewalk surfaces.
  - Avoid poorly lit parking lots at night.
  - Have your walking pattern evaluated if it is abnormal to see if an assistive device will help.
  - Practice balance-training, flexibility-training, and muscle-strengthening exercises.

GET INVOLVED IN A THERAPEUTIC EXERCISE PROGRAM

- Weight-bearing (standing) aerobic exercise
- Postural training
- Progressive resistance training for strengthening of large-muscle groups first, then smaller muscles

- Balance training for injury and fall prevention
- Stretching for flexibility to help reduce injuries and falls

CONSIDER JOINING A LOCAL OSTEOPOROSIS SUPPORT GROUP

Many patients with serious osteoporosis-related fractures experience some loss of independence. Their social roles may change, and they may feel isolated and suffer from depression. While medication and psychotherapy may be required to treat depression, other symptoms may be helped by the social interactions and educational programs in good support groups. If your doctor does not know about any of these groups, contact the National Osteoporosis Foundation (NOF; 202-223-2226) or the Department of Health in your state to see if they can help you find one in your area. In New York, contact the New York State Osteoporosis Prevention and Education Programs (NYSOPEP) for more information about NY support groups (845-786-4772). If you don't have a nearby support group, ask the NOF how to help initiate one.

THE BARE BONES

- Most acute fractures are initially evaluated and treated by an orthopedist, with some requiring casts and others requiring surgery.
- Most vertebral fractures are treated medically, initially with pain medicine, muscle relaxants, heat treatments, and sometimes back braces. Light activity is preferred to total bed rest; once the pain begins to subside, a set of exercises to train proper posture and strengthen the back muscles is

recommended. For people with severe persistent pain several weeks after a new vertebral fracture, vertebroplasty or kyphoplasty can be considered.

- Physical therapy may help patients get back on their feet, reduce pain faster, and help prevent future fractures.

- It is critical to realize that many fractures occurring in the absence of a major trauma such as a car accident are related to osteoporosis. Diagnosis of the underlying disease using bone density testing and medical treatment to prevent further deterioration and reduce the risk of future fractures is usually required.

- If you have had osteoporosis-related fractures, particularly of the spine or hip, ask your doctor if an outpatient or inpatient rehabilitation program or physical therapy program is appropriate for you.

- You should practice safe movement during all activities of daily living, keeping your back straight and avoiding forward bending.

- Review your home for safety to avoid falls.

- Engage in regular exercise to reduce pain, improve muscle and bone strength, and increase flexibility, thereby avoiding falls and future fracture.

- Ask your doctor whether you need a back support, hip protectors, or assistive devices for activities of daily living—or ask for a referral to a physical therapist to help make this decision.

- Look for an osteoporosis support group in your area.

Chapter 13

Medication for Osteoporosis in Women

This chapter outlines the groups of women who should and should not receive medication for osteoporosis, and briefly outlines the medications available for osteoporosis treatment.

While everyone should follow the prevention measures outlined in part II of this book, not everyone needs medication for osteoporosis. The choice ultimately depends on the likelihood of a person sustaining an osteoporosis-related fracture. While nobody has a crystal ball and our ability to predict the likelihood of fracturing is imperfect, we do have a lot of information about the factors known to increase the risk of fracture. The most logical way to determine who should receive medication for osteoporosis treatment, or fracture prevention, is to calculate the fracture risk and determine—based on reasonable clinical judgment regarding risks and benefits, as well as cost-effectiveness—what level of risk warrants pharmacologic intervention. In my opinion, for example, a woman who has approximately a 15 percent chance or higher of having a fracture related to osteoporosis over the next five years of her life should be treated. In some circumstances, I might recommend treatment for an even lower risk. The whole concept of absolute fracture risk, what should be used to calculate it, and what level of risk justifies treatment is still evolving.

It is critical that we set these risk guidelines to determine who should have therapy, since the benefit-to-cost ratio is not in favor of medicating those individuals at very low risk of fracturing. The cost I am referring to here is not only economic but also the burden of side effects and the psychological impact of taking medicine without a disease and with low risk of developing the disease. In the current world, where medications to prevent diseases are becoming increasingly common, we need to set reasonable limits on who should be treated.

It's worthwhile to divert a minute to consider how incredible it is that we now have medications that can reduce risk of chronic diseases. We've all accepted that when we have a disease, we may need a medication. Serious infections from bacteria should be treated with antibiotics, cancers may be treated with chemotherapy, and diseases such as lupus should be treated with immunosuppressant drugs. The idea that we can take drugs to reduce heart attacks (statin drugs), fractures (discussed in detail in the next several chapters), and breast cancer (tamoxifen and raloxifene) is mind-boggling. This trend will only proliferate in the upcoming decades.

Some women do not accept the concept of taking medication to prevent disease, whereas others want to take all available medicines to reduce the likelihood of getting any disease. The bottom line is that we all need to be educated and reasonable consumers in making these decisions. Surely we cannot put every adult on all of these preventive medications when it is unlikely that the disease we're trying to prevent will occur. It may be far more likely that the person will have a side effect from the medicine. Even in the case of aspirin, a rather benign medicine, it may be far more likely that a low-risk person will experience a gastrointestinal bleed (a bleeding ulcer, for example) than a heart attack. All of us should follow the preventive measures with regard to nutrition, exercise, and other lifestyle choices to maintain our health. Only people at elevated risk should consider a medicine to prevent the specific disease for which they are at increased risk.

WHO SHOULD RECEIVE TREATMENT?

It is clear that any woman who has had a hip fracture or a vertebral fracture in the absence of major trauma should be treated for osteoporosis. The risk of future fractures of both the spine and other sites is so high that treatment is justified in all such people.

One problem with this principle of treating all women who have had spine fractures is that people often do not know that they have had one, since they can occur without any presenting signs. Up until very recently, the only way to diagnose them was by obtaining a spine X ray. Since this is not a screening procedure and is not recommended in the absence of certain back symptoms (pain, deformity, substantial height loss), it is likely that we have incomplete information about one of the most important predictors of future fracture risk. Many vertebral compression deformities (which were previously undiagnosed) can now be seen on a specialized DXA image (lateral or instant vertebral assessment) at the time of BMD testing; in the near future, this may become a routine assessment done at the time of BMD testing. These measurements, additional to the bone density test, can prevent the extra time and radiation exposure associated with doing a spine X ray and, most importantly, will be able to pick up deformities that were previously not noted. These compression deformities are very strong predictors of the risk of new vertebral compressions, as well as other osteoporosis-related fractures. Therefore, these new procedures should be able to find additional women who should receive osteoporosis medication.

Aside from spine and hip fractures, we rely on the bone density measurement as well as a few clinical risk factors to determine who should be on medication for osteoporosis. We know that women who have a bone density T-Score in the osteoporosis range (–2.5) should all be treated.

T-Scores above –1 are completely normal and do not require further intervention. A person who has this level of T-Score should follow preventive measures and perhaps have the bone density repeated at some future date, but does not need therapy for protection against bone disease unless there are multiple serious risk factors present.

Levels in the lower part of the osteopenia range might be a harbinger of future osteoporosis and sometimes need to be treated, particularly if risk factors are present (see chapter 9). If no risk factors are present, it is usually not necessary to treat people with medicines in this range unless the levels are between –2 and –2.5. An exception to this guideline might be advanced age. Women in their midseventies, for example, might benefit from treatment even if the BMD is above –2.5. Age is probably the strongest risk factor for osteoporosis-related fracture besides BMD. For instance, a fifty-year-old woman with a T-Score of –2 (in the absence of other risk factors) has a five-year fracture probability of less than 10 percent whereas a seventy-year-old woman with the same bone mass could have a five-year risk of having a fracture of over 20 percent.

The other risk factors to consider in determining if a

woman in the osteopenia range needs medication are weight and any prior fractures. Weight is another important predictor of absolute fracture risk—lower weight is associated with higher risk of fracture, particularly of the hip. Weight less than 127 pounds doubles your risk of hip fracture compared to people who weigh more. Another very strong predictor of fracture risk is having a prior osteoporosis-related fracture. Further risk factors that might justify treatment at a higher BMD level include a family history of osteoporosis-related fracture and current or very recent smoking history.

Someday in the near future we will have an ability to incorporate much of this information into the bone density testing and reporting process in order to calculate each individual's absolute risk of having an osteoporosis-related fracture.

WHAT ARE THE MEDICATION CHOICES?

Once it is determined that medication is necessary, the decision about which medication should be taken must be made. The choices of medicines that are approved by the U.S. Food and Drug Administration for the prevention and/or treatment of osteoporosis include:

- Hormone or estrogen therapies (see chapter 14)
- Raloxifene (Evista)
- Alendronate (Fosamax)
- Risedronate (Actonel)
- Calcitonin nasal spray (Miacalcin)
- Parathyroid hormone (PTH or Forteo)

In the next several chapters of this book, I will describe the different medications with their benefits and risks, as well as providing some reasonable framework as to how to determine when and if to use a specific drug. The hormone or estrogen therapies, as well as raloxifene, are all agents that have effects throughout the body, and these will all be briefly reviewed. The other agents are bone-specific, meaning that although they may produce an occasional side effect, they do not exert substantial effects in areas other than the skeleton. The medication called tamoxifen will also be discussed in chapter 15 on Selective Estrogen Receptor Modulators (SERMS), because it is used in many postmenopausal women for treatment and prevention of breast cancer and may have beneficial effects on the skeleton.

Other medicines are available in pharmacies for other diseases and may be used with some success in osteoporosis. There are good clinical research studies for some of these compounds, although they are sometimes not approved because the manufacturer does not wish to obtain an indication specifically for osteoporosis, or because the FDA does not believe that there is enough data to support the efficacy of the medication for the osteoporosis indication. The medicines that are most likely to be used in this fashion are best used as last resorts when approved medicines are not tolerated or are contraindicated. These other medications will be discussed in chapter 19.

THE BARE BONES

- If you are considering taking a medication for osteoporosis, you should follow the universal prevention measures, including reducing risk factors, optimizing nutrition, and getting regular exercise.

- If you have had vertebral or hip fractures, you are at high risk for future fractures and need medication in addition to prevention measures.
- If your bone density test indicates that you have osteoporosis, you should receive medication.
- If you have a borderline bone density score (between −1.5 and −2.5) your doctor should review your clinical risk factors (age, personal fracture history, family medical history, and so forth) and should consider initiating treatment depending on the number and severity of these factors in addition to the degree of osteopenia.
- You must consider the benefits and risks of each agent in discussion with your doctor to determine which medication, if any, is right for you.
- No medication could ever be available or approved for osteoporosis or any other disease without people willing to participate in randomized controlled clinical trials.

Chapter 14

Estrogen or Hormone Therapy

CASE STUDY

A fifty-one-year-old woman had her last menstrual period about six months ago. Ever since her menstrual periods became irregular, about a year before that, she had been plagued by hot flashes and night sweats that prevented her from getting a decent night's sleep. Several months ago, she slipped on a patch of ice on her driveway, fell, and broke her wrist. It was casted and healed well. Her gynecologist suggested a bone density test, which indicated a T-Score of –2 in the lumbar spine and –2.4 in the hip region. There is no family or personal history of phlebitis or breast disease, and she has no cardiac disease risk factors.

This patient clearly needs treatment for osteoporosis and is a good candidate for estrogen treatment. It will relieve her hot flashes and at the same time prevent bone loss and reduce the risk of more fractures. She should plan on a few years of estrogen and then look at other effective treatment options.

This chapter reviews the complex issues of estrogen and hormone therapy and tries to provide some perspective on how our concepts of these medications have changed over the years. Both the skeletal and nonskeletal effects are discussed, and results from the recently stopped part of the Women's Health Initiative are highlighted.

There is a movement in the field to change the term "replacement therapy" to "therapy" since these hormones are not normally present in postmenopausal women. Therefore we are not actually "replacing." Throughout this chapter, I will refer to ET and HT as estrogen therapy and hormone therapy.

Estrogens are hormones produced principally by the ovaries. In addition to their effects on the reproductive system (the initiation of puberty, from breast development to normal menstrual function—as well as during pregnancy), estrogens are important in the maintenance of normal healthy bone and bone metabolism. Bones are normally undergoing a continuous remodeling process in which old bone is removed and replaced with new bone. Loss of estrogen at any age results in an increase in the rate of this remodeling process and an imbalance between the destruction and formation phases of remodeling, such that more bone is removed than is replaced. If you magnify this imbalance by initiating many of these remodeling sites throughout the skeleton at one time, a measurable amount of bone loss will occur. Therefore, estrogen loss at menopause— or before—is associated with loss of bone and an increase in the risk of all fractures.

It has long been known that estrogen intervention, often called estrogen replacement therapy (ERT or ET) or hormone replacement therapy (HRT or HT), returns the bone remodeling rate to the healthy low levels seen in normally menstruating younger women. While we do not know that these premenopausal rates of bone remodeling are actually the optimal levels, we believe them to be, because bone mass is relatively stable and fracture rates are the lowest at that stage in life. In fact, all the agents currently available for osteoporosis treatment, except PTH (see chapter 18), work by reducing rates of bone resorption and remodeling. In so doing, estrogen prevents bone loss. Furthermore, the results of the massive study known as the Women's Health Initiative (WHI) confirm that HT does reduce the risk of osteoporosis-related fracture.

The Food and Drug Administration has approved a number of estrogens for use in the prevention of osteoporosis. Others are approved specifically for management of menopausal symptoms (such as hot flashes), but may be used for osteoporosis prevention as well. A list of various estrogens, progestins, and estrogen plus progestin combinations currently available is shown in figure 14-1.

Estrogens, Progestins and Combination Products

Estrogen Pills

Premarin	conjugated equine estrogens
Cenestin	synthetic conjugated estrogens
Estratab	esterified estrogens
Menest	esterified estrogens
Ortho-Est	estropipate (piperazine estrone sulfate)
Estrace	micronized 17-beta-estradiol

Estrogen Skin Patch

Alora	micronized 17-beta-estradiol
Climara	micronized 17-beta-estradiol
Esclim	micronized 17-beta-estradiol
Estraderm	micronized 17-beta-estradiol
Vivelle	micronized 17-beta-estradiol
Vivelle-Dot	micronized 17-beta-estradiol

Progestin Pills

Amen	medroxyprogesterone acetate
Cyrin	medroxyprogesterone acetate
Provera	medroxyprogesterone acetate
Micronor	norethindrone
Nor-QD	norethindrone
Aygestin	norethindrone acetate
Ovrette	norgestrel
Norplant	levonorgestrel
Prometrium	progesterone USP
Megace	megestrol acetate

Estrogen Plus Progestin Pills

Premphase	conjugated equine estrogens and medroxyprogesterone acetate
Prempro	conjugated equine estrogens and medroxyprogesterone acetate
Femhrt	ethinylestradiol and norethindrone acetate
Activella	17-beta-estradiol and norethindrone acetate
Ortho-Prefest	17-beta-estradiol and norethindrone acetate

Estrogen Plus Progestin Skin Patches

Combipatch	17-beta-estradiol and norethindrone acetate
Ortho-Prefest	17-beta-estradiol and norethindrone

Table 14-1.

SKELETAL EFFECTS

A large body of well-performed controlled studies (in which women are randomly assigned to receive estrogens or sugar pills; see appendix A) from many centers throughout the United States and Europe confirms that ET and HT can maintain or increase bone mass throughout the skeleton. This is true in both healthy early postmenopausal women and in older women with and without osteoporosis. The greatest effects are usually seen in the spine, but bone mass of any measured site, including the hand, wrist, hip, and total body, can be shown to improve with estrogen therapy. Greater effects on bone density are seen when ET or HT are combined with adequate calcium intake.

In general, the benefits of therapy to bone mass decline with time after discontinuing therapy. In fact, there appears to be a particularly rapid loss of bone in the first few years after stopping ET or HT. Therefore, five to ten years after stopping treatment, bone density values may be indistinguishable from those of women who have never taken estrogen.

Over the last five years, studies have shown that lower doses of estrogen (for example, 0.3 mg conjugated estrogens instead of 0.625 mg) are also effective at maintaining or slightly increasing bone mass. Most, but not all, studies indicate that the use of HT in which progestin (another hormone produced by the ovary) is added to protect the uterus from abnormal growth and increased risk of uterine cancer probably does not have a meaningful effect on bone density separate from the effect of estrogen itself (see the end of this chapter).

One of the confusing concepts about bone mass and fractures is that there is no guarantee that a change in bone density with medication will definitely reduce fracture occurrence throughout the body. This is despite the proven fact that bone mass in an untreated woman is an excellent predictor of the risk of fracture and the only way to diagnose osteoporosis before a fracture occurs. But the amount of increase in bone mass with medication doesn't relate that well to the amount of protection against fracture. Only small changes in bone mass seem to be required with various osteoporosis medications to result in a reduction in risk of spine fracture. This may not be true of fractures in other parts of the skeleton; we simply do not know at this point, since only two types of medications (HT and bis-phosphonates, chapter 17) have been clearly proven to reduce the occurrence of hip fracture—and both produce substantial, similar, increments in bone mass. Therefore—as with all osteoporosis medications—*it is imperative to prove that a medication works to reduce fractures in order to recommend its use for osteoporosis treatment.* When it comes to osteoporosis prevention, we only have to show that the medicine prevents bone loss.

Until the WHI results were published, only a few randomized clinical trials had evaluated fracture occurrence with ET or HT. Taken together, these small studies suggested that ET and HT could reduce the risk of spine and nonspine fractures. These earlier trials were consistent with the large number of observational studies (see appendix A for a description of observational studies) showing that ET or HT, given to postmenopausal women for at least five years, is associated with a reduction in the risk of fractures. The observational data indicated a decrease in the risk of hip and other fractures by as much as 50 percent.

Until the WHI was published, however, there was no randomized controlled trial confirming that estrogens could really reduce the risk of hip fracture. In contrast, the largest randomized trial of HT before WHI—called the Heart & Estrogen/Progestin Study (HERS) conducted in more than 2,700 patients with established heart disease—did not show a reduction in hip or any other clinical osteoporotic fractures. However, this study evaluated the effect of HT started in an older group of women (average age sixty-six), who already had heart disease and who were not chosen for high risk of osteoporosis. In fact, less than 15 percent of the women in the study had osteoporosis. It is more difficult to demonstrate an effect of any medication against fracture occurrence in people at low risk.

Therefore, the results of this one important clinical trial do not negate the consensus of data from observational studies and the other available randomized clinical studies.

In contrast to the findings of HERS, the results of the WHI confirm the other few randomized controlled trials and the overwhelmingly positive observational studies of HRT/ERT use and fracture occurrence. The WHI enrolled more than 16,600 postmenopausal women between the ages of fifty and seventy-nine into a study of daily HT (Prempro) versus placebo. Although the study was planned to continue for eight and a half years, it was terminated early due to safety concerns. The study was gratifying in terms of its conclusions about fractures. WHI showed that HT produced a 34 percent reduction in hip fracture risk, a 34 percent reduction in symptomatic vertebral fractures, and a 24 percent reduction in all osteoporosis-related fractures. Therefore, the knowledge about estrogen's role in the physiology of menopause-related bone loss, and the effects of estrogen replacement on bone remodeling, bone mass, and fracture reduction are all consistent.

ESTROGEN ADMINISTRATION

The most widely used daily form is 0.625 mg conjugated equine estrogen (Premarin), but many other estrogens are available in pill or patch form (see figure 14-1 on page 167). Recent studies have shown that lower-dose estrogens protect effectively against bone loss as well.

Estrogen regimens are usually prescribed continuously (every day of the month), but short periods off ET may be useful if breast tenderness is a problem. If the uterus is present, a progestin (progesterone) must be given to prevent thickening of the lining of the uterus and thus avoid increasing the risk of uterine cancer. The progestin part of the hormone regimen can be given daily or for twelve days each month. In the former regimen, patients can avoid menstrual-type bleeding, but in the latter, bleeding often occurs as the progestin is finished. Combination pills and skin patches of estrogen and progestin are also available.

Progestins need not be used in the absence of a uterus. These agents alone are less effective than estrogens and should not be used as sole agents in the maintenance of health after menopause or in the prevention or treatment of osteoporosis per se. They may be associated with more side effects than estrogens. Furthermore, there is evidence now that progestins may increase the risk of breast cancer. In studies comparing regimens that combine estrogen and progestin with the use of estrogens alone, the risk of breast cancer is substantially higher with combinations. Whether this is a function of the progestin alone or of the two hormones somehow working together cannot be determined from the available data. Still, I believe it prudent to use the lowest possible dose of progestin and not to opt for progestin alone as a hormonal treatment of choice.

EFFECTS THROUGHOUT THE BODY

Vascular Disease

Epidemiological data indicate that premenopausal women have lower rates of heart disease than age-matched postmenopausal women. Observational studies suggest that estrogens (both alone and with progestins) reduce the risk of heart disease. Many controlled trials indicate that estrogens produce benefits on intermediate markers of heart health, such as cholesterol. In fact, for many years, many of us were prescribing estrogens to reduce heart disease. Despite all these findings, however, there have been no controlled clinical trials confirming that estrogens, either alone or with progestins, reduce the risk of heart disease. In contrast, the HERS clinical trial revealed that patients who had preexisting cardiac disease, and were assigned to HT, did not reduce the overall likelihood of cardiovascular disease (such as heart attack, surgical procedure, or hospitalization) over four years. In fact, the risk of heart disease was actually increased in the first year among HT users in this study. These results were corroborated by a number of other clinical trials evaluating the benefit of various estrogens and estrogen/progestin combinations on the risk of heart disease, stroke, and amount of plaque buildup in coronary arteries. The studies have consistently showed lack of benefit in reducing risk of disease progression.

Until the WHI, it was argued that the results of ET/HT on heart disease might differ in a younger population of women who do not yet have known disease (called primary prevention, rather than secondary prevention). However, the results of the Women's Health Initiative indicate that even in women without known heart disease, there is no protective effect of HT; in fact, similar to the HERS trial, there was an increase in risk of both heart attack (risk increased 29 percent) and stroke (risk increased 41 percent).

Based on what we know now, ET or HT should not be started in women with known heart disease or stroke disease and probably those known to be at high risk for developing it. The American Heart Association has recently come out with a policy statement with this basic conclusion. There are other extremely effective modalities for prevention of vascular disease, which should be considered in anyone at significant risk, including aspirin and statin drugs.

Why do the results of the WHI clinical trial differ so much from the observational studies with regard to heart disease? One reason has to do with the difference between randomized clinical trials and observational studies. As discussed in detail in appendix A, randomized trials feature study groups and control groups designed to have similar characteristics (age, risk factors, medication usage, weight, and general health among others). In observational studies, the study group chooses to take the medication, and is then compared with a group of people who choose not to. The comparison group is usually similar in terms of age, but many other characteristics may be different between the two groups. Both groups are followed over time to determine what diseases they develop. Since women select whether to take medication or not, there may be other factors influencing the results. The two groups may not be well matched in terms of important health characteristics. Therefore, in the modern world where we are asking for proof that medicines really work, the randomized clinical trial stands out as the best type of study.

There appear to be differences between people who use estrogen and those who do not with regard to educational level, socioeconomic class, other health issues, nutrition, exercise, and other factors. It may be one or more of these other factors that produces the apparent association between estrogen use and reduced heart disease. In fact, recent analyses of all of the observational studies of HT and heart disease that took differences in socioeconomic status into account showed no reductions in heart disease.

Cancer

Estrogens prescribed without progestins increase the risk of uterine cancer. Therefore, all women who have not had a hysterectomy must take a progestin with estrogen. There are many different progestins, and it is not clear which is the best. Micronized progesterone may have some advantages over older, more traditional forms such as medroxyprogesterone acetate in terms of side effects and effects on blood cholesterol levels. Progestin is best administered in pill form; creams offer unreliable absorption and unproven effectiveness at reducing risk of uterine cancer in combination with estrogen.

Epidemiologic studies show that long-term estrogen use (more than five to ten years) is associated with an increase in the risk of breast cancer, especially among thin women. There was never any evidence to suggest a reduction in the increased risk of breast cancer when progestins are also used. In fact, progestins added to estrogen probably increase breast cancer risk compared to estrogens alone.

The WHI has now confirmed that HT (Prempro) is associated with an increase in the risk of breast cancer of about 26 percent. The increased breast cancer risk begins to be apparent after about four years of use. It is not yet known whether unopposed estrogen (without progestins) given to women without a uterus also results in increased risk of breast cancer. The part of the WHI that is studying estrogen alone is still going on. This must mean that some of the risks associated with HT are not seen with ET alone, or that the benefits are greater. Perhaps we will have more information shortly after this book is published.

A mammogram is required before starting an estrogen regimen. Furthermore, regular physical examination of the breast (monthly self-examination and once- or twice-yearly examination by a physician) and annual mammography are critically important for women on estrogens. These recommendations are consistent with the National Cancer Institute's recommendations for this age group even when estrogen is not used.

Recent new large observational studies show that estrogens taken without progestins for longer than ten years may also be associated with an increased risk of ovarian cancer. In the case of the ovary, progestins might be protective in reducing or eliminating this risk. The ovary and the uterus are the two areas where progestins may actually be exerting a beneficial effect, instead of a negative one. Still, statistically, ovarian cancer is so much less common than breast cancer that it is reasonable to avoid taking progestins if you have had a hysterectomy. Moreover, the unopposed ET arm of the WHI might help us evaluate this issue.

It may be that new and evolving products, such as progestins delivered through a vaginal ring around the cervix, can deliver progestins to the organs for which a benefit is seen (uterus and ovary) while systemic general absorption of the medication is limited. This may avoid the detrimental effects while maintaining the beneficial ones.

Observational studies have shown that ET/HT use for longer than five years appears to be associated with a decrease in the risk of colon cancer. The WHI has now confirmed that HT can reduce the risk of colorectal cancer by a magnitude of 37 percent. The relative benefit of HT for this purpose needs to be weighed against the risks and considered in light of other agents that may also have preventive actions against colorectal cancer, such as calcium and aspirin.

Other Effects

Estrogens are extremely effective in reducing symptoms of menopause, especially hot flashes, night sweats, and insomnia as well as vaginal dryness and itching. Since estrogens increase the risk of gallbladder disease, symptoms of upper abdominal pain and/or nausea should be investigated to rule out gallstones. A link between an increase in the risk of blood clots in veins (phlebitis) and ET has also been established. The WHI proved that HT increases the risk of these blood clots by more than 100 percent.

Preliminary data suggesting a relationship between declining estrogen levels at menopause with memory loss and Alzheimer's disease, and the ability of ET or HT to reduce these effects, needs to be confirmed with more clinical trial data. At the moment, it would not be reasonable to begin HT for this purpose. Furthermore, the influence of estrogen on reducing urinary incontinence or pelvic organ prolapse has not been firmly established.

REMAINING QUESTIONS ABOUT HT

We do not know if the results of WHI extend to all estrogen/progesterone preparations. Not all estrogens are equivalent, and not all progestins are equivalent. There have been no large-scale clinical trials evaluating estrogen/progestin combinations other than Prempro, and it is unlikely that large clinical studies with other hormone combinations will be done. In lieu of any information otherwise, it is probably reasonable to consider that other HT regimens produce similar risks and benefits to Prempro. Furthermore, it is unknown whether treatment with estrogen alone (Premarin) will produce the same risks and benefits or same magnitude of these effects as HT (Prempro). Since the unopposed arm of the WHI is still ongoing, it is likely that there will be some differences between Premarin and Prempro. The risk-to-benefit ratio for recently postmenopausal women is not yet established since no subgroup analysis for this young select group has been presented or published. This is the group of women for whom HT is most likely going to be recommended.

REACTIONS TO THE WHI NEWS

In women who are in their forties who had a very early menopause, or for women in their early fifties on HT for only a short time, I have continued HT with the plan to stop it in a few years. I don't think the WHI results apply to these patients. Many of my other patients had already been thinking about stopping their estrogens because I had prepared them with the idea that after five to ten years of therapy, I would recommend discontinuing treatment. This policy was based solely on the basis of increasing risk of breast cancer. These patients were happy to use the WHI news as the time to make the change. Many women have tolerated a tapering of the estrogen dose over weeks to months with few symptoms. In my experience, suddenly stopping estrogens is more likely to produce symptoms. A few women have had lots of difficulty with hot flashes even during the tapering and withdrawal of estrogens. In a few of these cases, the estrogens have been restarted at low dose; some of these women have tried different hormone regimens, while some have elected to restart their Prempro.

In some women, I have recommended alternatives for hot flashes with success. The commonly used class of antidepressants, the SSRIs, has been shown to reduce hot flashes. The one with the most data is venlafaxine (Effexor). Some women, even those well within the range studied in the WHI study, still feel comfortable remaining on HT. It is important in this regard to realize that the absolute risks are not that high. One perspective, for example, is to consider the excess cases produced by the HT, compared to the baseline risk (see figure 14-2). For every 10,000 women treated with Prempro for 1 year, there will be 7 excess heart attacks, 8 excess strokes, 8 excess breast cancer cases, and 18 extra venous thromboembolic events (blood clots in veins or lungs); there will also be 6 fewer cases of colon cancer and 5 fewer hip fractures. These numbers might seem rather small but should be magnified by the number of years of use.

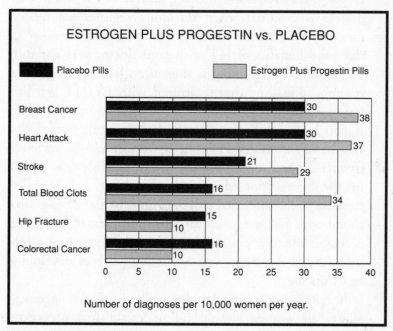

Figure 14-2: This data indicates higher rates of certain medical conditions, such as blood clots and breast cancer, in women on estrogen plus progestin pills.

THE BARE BONES

- The only real surprise in the WHI results was the increased heart disease and stroke risks. The increased risk of breast cancer and protection against fracture and colon cancer were all expected based on prior observational studies.

- The WHI was stopped after only five of the planned eight-plus years because the increased risks of heart disease (29 percent), stroke (41 percent), and breast cancer (26 percent) outweighed the reduced risks of hip fracture (34 percent) and colorectal cancer (37 percent).

- A discussion about the multiple benefits and risks of estrogen use in relation to your own individual risk of each disease is essential when hormone regimes are recommended to women. Furthermore, you must review the risks and benefits of HT with your doctor very carefully every six to twelve months thereafter. It is no longer reasonable to assume that treatment with ET/HT is a lifelong proposition.

- If you have debilitating hot flashes or night sweats, you should still consider HT, but its use should be reviewed frequently. You should use the lowest possible dose of HT for the shortest possible period of time.

- Because of the increased risk of cardiovascular disease associated with HT use, even early in the treatment period, it is reasonable to avoid initiating therapy if you have established heart disease or you are at high risk of developing heart disease.

- It is critical to realize that for osteoporosis management alone, all women should follow established preventive measures (nutrition, exercise, and lifestyle)—and that if medication is needed, there are a number of effective alternatives to HT. A full discussion of those alternatives, including raloxifene, alendronate, risedronate, calcitonin, and PTH, is essential if your primary goal with HT is osteoporosis prevention and/or treatment.

Chapter 15

Selective Estrogen Receptor Modulators

CASE STUDY

A fifty-five-year-old healthy woman with no prior fractures had her last menstrual period about four years earlier. She took estrogens for several months for hot flashes but stopped over three years before. A bone density test done for routine screening purposes showed her spine T-score to be –2.3 with a hip T-score of –1.3. Her mother had a stooped posture and was diagnosed with breast cancer in her sixties. This woman would benefit from raloxifene (Evista) to protect her bone mass and help prevent spine fractures. She might also derive a benefit against breast cancer.

The name for drugs in this class—selective estrogen receptor modulators, or SERMs—derives from the fact that they bind to the estrogen receptor. Despite this, though, they are not considered estrogens because their chemical structures differ. The different shape of these agents when they bind to the estrogen receptors in different cells produces different effects from those of estrogen. These medications produce some effects that are similar to those of estrogen in some tissues and opposite to those of estrogens in others. As a class, these agents seem to avoid stimulating the breast tissue, and in fact at least raloxifene and tamoxifen appear to reduce the risk of developing breast cancer. These medications are both used in postmenopausal women, for different reasons. Raloxifene or Evista is FDA-approved for the prevention and treatment of osteoporosis. Tamoxifen or Nolvadex is approved for the treatment and prevention of breast cancer.

TAMOXIFEN

When tamoxifen was first introduced as a treatment for breast cancer in all different stages of the disease, it was expected that the skeleton might suffer adverse consequences from the drug. The fact that it acted as an estrogen-blocking agent on breast tissue seemed to imply that it would act that way on the bones also and produce loss of bone tissue. Instead it was found to actually help preserve bone, at least in the spine, and later also demonstrated to preserve bone in the hip. It turned out that tamoxifen was acting opposite to estrogen on the breast and like estrogen on the bone. Now we see that this class of drugs can have tissue-specific effects, with each of the agents having its own profile in terms of whether its effect is estrogenlike or estrogen-blocking in each specific part of the body.

Although tamoxifen does preserve bone in postmenopausal women who have a history of breast cancer (and also those who do not have a prior history), it appears to have estrogen-blocking activity in premenopausal women in the skeleton. This is an important distinction since tamoxifen is now approved for both treatment and prevention of breast cancer in premenopausal and postmenopausal women. It might very well have a different risk-to-benefit ratio in premenopausal women.

As discussed in chapter 14, because the relationship between increases in bone mass with medications and fracture reduction effectiveness is not that strong, it is important to look at the occurrence of fractures in women on any medication thought to have an effect on bone, including tamoxifen. Here the number of studies to review is very limited. There is one good clinical investigation of tamoxifen in women who were enrolled in a Breast Cancer Prevention Trial called BCPT. The 13,388 women in this randomized controlled trial (see appendix A for description) had no prior history of breast cancer but were thought to be at increased risk on the basis of age greater than sixty, or other risk factors such as family history of breast cancer, having no children, previous breast biopsies, previously abnormal tissue on a breast biopsy (but not true cancer), and others. Here the number of fractures of the spine, hip, and wrist was modestly lower in the women assigned to tamoxifen, but the reduction in frequency was not statistically significant. Also, the total number of all fractures was about the same in tamoxifen-treated as placebo-treated women. Therefore, the study was not totally convincing that tamoxifen could reduce fracture occurrence. This is not unexpected, since the study included many premenopausal women, and even the postmenopausal women might have been at low risk of osteoporosis-related fracture. It is often difficult to demonstrate a reduction in fracture in people who are at low risk of osteoporosis.

Nevertheless, because of the uncertainty about tamoxifen and its role in the reduction of fractures and because the drug is probably not as potent as other bone-specific medications, it is probably reasonable to consider a medication specific for osteoporosis (such as a bisphosphonate) in women who are on tamoxifen for prevention or treatment of breast cancer and who have osteoporosis by bone density or fracture criteria. This is probably also a consideration for women who have borderline bone mass and who are losing bone mass on serial bone density measurements. In contrast, for women who are on tamoxifen and do not have osteoporosis, it is reasonable to avoid starting another treatment and consider the tamoxifen a preventive treatment against bone loss.

Tamoxifen is not used as frequently as suggested by the FDA indications for prevention of breast cancer. In part, this is because many women do not realize that there actually is a medication that can prevent breast cancer. Also, many women do not wish to take a medication, even if it does prevent disease. The same is true of medication for osteoporosis. We recommend treatment for women at high risk of fractures who have no current symptoms of any disease, to prevent fractures and their associated symptoms from developing. Furthermore, like all drugs, tamoxifen can produce certain side effects. These include an increase in the risk of cancer of the lining of the uterus (endometrial or uterine cancer). Although the baseline risk of this disease is rather low, the increase in risk attributable to tamoxifen is substantial—three to five or more times increased. Tamoxifen also stimulates growth of benign uterine tissue and can cause vaginal bleeding from fibroids or benign uterine lining thickening. The other possible risks are blood clots in the veins of the legs (deep vein thrombosis), which can sometimes break off and travel to the lungs (pulmonary embolism). These complications are very serious, usually requiring hospitalization followed by blood-thinning medication for many months. Tamoxifen can also increase the development of cataracts and need for cataract surgery. It can also produce less serious side effects that can be very bothersome, such as hot flashes.

RALOXIFENE

Raloxifene was developed for osteoporosis. It was shown to prevent bone loss and actually increase bone mass modestly at all sites in healthy postmenopausal women. These were women who had slightly reduced bone mass compared to young normal women (T-Scores of −1 to −2.5) but were all above the osteoporosis range. In general, prevention studies are designed to look at effects on bone mass alone. In prevention populations, bone mass is only slightly reduced and fracture risk is not particularly high. As a result, a study in this population would have to be outrageously large or prohibitively long in order to determine if the effects on bone mass could also translate into effects on fracture occurrence.

A separate large randomized clinical trial called MORE (Multiple Outcomes of Raloxifene Evaluation) was performed to determine if raloxifene could be effective at reducing fracture occurrence in women who already had osteoporosis (where fracture risk is high enough to see the effect). The osteoporosis treatment study was well designed, rigorous, and very large—enrolling more than 7,700 women with osteoporosis. Some of these women had vertebral fractures, and others had osteoporosis defined by bone density alone. Raloxifene increased bone mass moderately in all sites (2 to 3 percent compared to the bone mass levels in the placebo control group at the spine, hip, and wrist). It reduced the occurrence of vertebral fractures (deformities diagnosed by X ray) by 35 to 50 percent (with slight differences in various subgroups) over four years of treatment. There was no clear reduction in risk of fractures at other parts of the body, however. For example, hip, wrist, and all nonvertebral fractures did not occur less frequently in women assigned to raloxifene.

We do not have a good explanation for why a medication could work so well for one type of fracture but not for another. One possible explanation is that there are different types of bone predominant in the spine compared to the hip and limb bones in general. The spine is composed primarily of cancellous or spongy bone, which looks like a lacy lattice with magnification. The hip, arms, and legs are composed primarily of cortical or compact bone, which is much denser and less metabolically active. We believe that the greater magnitude of increase in bone mass of the spine, compared to all other skeletal sites, when osteoporosis medication is administered, is related to the predominance of cancellous bone. It may be that the bone mass change is not big enough at the hip or other sites compared to that at the spine. There are differences in the mechanical forces that cross the hip compared to those that cross the spine. The bone shapes are very different, and it may be more difficult to effect a big change in hip strength. Certainly, it is clear that it is easier for a medication to reduce spine fractures than it is to reduce hip fractures.

Effects in Other Areas of the Body

Aside from working to improve bone mass throughout the skeleton—and reducing the occurrence of vertebral fractures by up to 50 percent over four years—raloxifene has effects on other areas of the body that are equally important. In contrast to tamoxifen, it does not increase the risk of uterine cancer; nor does it produce uterine thickening or polyps. As a result, there is no need to take a second hormone, progestin or progesterone, with raloxifene. Therefore, there should be no vaginal bleeding or spotting with raloxifene use.

Similar to tamoxifen, however, through the major osteoporosis treatment study mentioned above (MORE), we discovered that raloxifene could also reduce the risk of breast cancer. This finding is highly significant. Overall, raloxifene reduces breast cancer occurrence by about 70 percent. This may be even better than tamoxifen. The reduction is seen with breast tumors that are estrogen receptor positive, which is the case with the vast majority of the breast cancers seen in postmenopausal women. It is unclear whether raloxifene is actually preventing cancer cells from forming in the first place, or reducing the growth of cancer cells that have already formed. The rapid reduction seen in breast cancers that can be diagnosed clinically when raloxifene is administered argues for the latter. We know that cancer cells are generally alive for a long time before the tumor can grow enough to become noticeable or visible. It is possible that raloxifene could both reduce the growth of existing cells and kill off existing cells—or even prevent cancer cells from forming. These are distinctions that cannot be made from the existing data. Regardless, obviously it is a very beneficial effect, and it is equally compelling to its ability to reduce vertebral fractures from osteoporosis.

It is of historical interest that raloxifene many years ago was being investigated for its effectiveness on breast cancer. At that time, based on an extremely small study in thirteen patients with breast cancer who had already failed tamoxifen treatment, the development of raloxifene was abandoned. It was pulled off the shelf many years later after publication of some of the tamoxifen observations showing a beneficial effect on bone and subsequent confirmation obtained by studies in animal models of osteoporosis and estrogen deficiency. Now, many years later, it appears that the medication is useful for health of both bone and breast.

There is currently an ongoing large clinical trial called STAR (Study of Tamoxifen and Raloxifene), which plans to enroll about 20,000 women who are at increased risk of breast cancer. The intention of this randomized study is to compare breast cancer rates in tamoxifen- compared to raloxifene-treated women and to determine if one drug is superior to the other at suppressing clinically appearing breast tumors over a five-year period. The study will also compare the side effects and important safety factors between the two drugs. Other outcomes being evaluated include fractures. Data from this important study should be available in the second half of this decade. Until then, we cannot know with certainty which drug is better for breast cancer prevention. Given what we know now, though, despite the lack of FDA approval for raloxifene as a breast cancer preventive agent, many doctors are using it in this capacity.

Another important area evaluated in MORE is heart and vascular disease. Recent findings indicate there is no increase in risk of any circulatory problems of the heart and brain at any time over the course of raloxifene treatment in contrast to what is seen with HT. Moreover, in women who have established heart disease or who are at increased risk on the basis of a set of clinical risk factors, raloxifene appears to protect against the development of fatal and nonfatal heart attacks and angina as well as strokes and transient ischemic attacks. In women without prior disease or who were not at high risk of developing it, there was no statistically significant effect of raloxifene, in part because the rate of events was low, as expected. These findings are very encouraging and suggest that another important beneficial effect on health in some postmenopausal women may be seen with use of raloxifene.

The effects of raloxifene on heart disease, stroke, and breast cancer are being evaluated further in a large study called RUTH (Raloxifene Use in the Heart). This randomized controlled trial will compare the effect of raloxifene to placebo over seven years in more than 10,000 women who are at high risk of developing heart disease or stroke. This important study will determine for which patients, if any, it is reasonable to prescribe this medication to protect against these diseases. Heart disease remains the number one cause of death in women. The possibility of reducing the risk of three diseases—osteoporosis, breast cancer, and heart attacks or stroke—with one medication is obviously extremely appealing. The RUTH study will also provide more information on other possible outcomes of raloxifene, including fractures.

Two other areas are important to mention. Cognitive assessments have been performed in patients on placebo and on raloxifene. There were no significant differences in cognitive function between those patients who received placebo compared to those people who received raloxifene over the course of the study. Furthermore, there appeared to be no dramatic effect of raloxifene on risk of pelvic organ prolapse (bladder, uterus) or need for prolapse surgery; in fact, raloxifene appeared to reduce the risk of prolapse surgery. This was also an important finding from MORE, since over the last decade several other drugs in the SERM class that were under development for osteoporosis or other indications were determined to produce an increase in pelvic organ prolapse.

Side Effects

There is of course no drug completely without side effects. Raloxifene is generally very well tolerated and can be taken at any time of the day, with or without food. It can increase hot flashes in a small percentage of people. In general, we avoid giving raloxifene to early menopausal women who have hot flashes or night sweats because of this potential side effect. For unclear reasons, raloxifene can also produce leg cramps; some patients also retain fluid in the hands, feet, and legs. These side effects rarely are severe enough to induce people to stop the medication. An occasional side effect is that a person will feel systemically ill, as if she is developing a virus such as the flu. In the rare case when this occurs, the symptoms usually abate within about twenty-four hours of starting the medicine.

Only one serious adverse event has been seen with raloxifene: blood clots of the veins of the legs (phlebitis), retina (part of the eye), and/or the circulatory system of the lung. This is quite rare, and the risk is almost identical to that seen with estrogen or hormone therapy. One factor that must be discussed with your doctor before considering use of any SERM or hormonal agent such as raloxifene, tamoxifen, or estrogen is whether there is a previous personal or family history of phlebitis or any other clotting disorder. Patients who are immobilized or nonambulatory may also be at elevated risk for blood clots with raloxifene (or any SERM or estrogen). For this reason, it is recommended that you stop raloxifene for several days prior to elective surgery or a long car ride or flight. Aside from this clinical information, however, there really is not a great way to predict who is going to develop this serious side effect. There are some tests that, if positive, might be associated with an increased risk of clotting, but their predictive value at the current time is too low to be of good general clinical use: Too many patients who don't show positive will have the side effect and too many patients who do show positive on the test will not have the side effect.

THE BARE BONES

- Raloxifene and tamoxifen are not estrogens, but they do work in part through the estrogen receptor.
- Raloxifene protects against bone loss and fractures of the spine.
- Both tamoxifen and raloxifene appear to protect against breast cancer, but only tamoxifen is FDA-approved for this use. The relative magnitude of this effect and the relative safety of the drugs are currently being explored (STAR).
- In preliminary data, raloxifene appears to reduce the risk of heart disease and stroke in women who are at high risk. The potential protective benefit of raloxifene against cardiovascular disease is being studied further in a large clinical trial called RUTH.
- While tamoxifen can increase the risk of uterine cancer, raloxifene does not.
- Both raloxifene and tamoxifen (as well as estrogen) increase risk of venous blood clots, but these are rare in healthy women.

Chapter 16

Calcitonin

CASE STUDY

Recently, a seventy-eight-year-old woman felt severe sudden back pain while vacuuming her living room. An X ray ordered in the emergency room showed a compression fracture due to osteoporosis. The woman was healthy aside from a stricture of the esophagus making it impossible to take Fosamax or Actonel. She was given Miacalcin to help her with the pain and to help stabilize her situation. She was also referred to a specialist to review her other options, including trying the new bone-building drug Forteo, or participating in a clinical trial.

Calcitonin is a small protein hormone normally produced in the thyroid gland. It is totally distinct from thyroid hormone, also produced by the thyroid gland. While the function of thyroid hormone is very clear, and without it sickness and death result, the function of calcitonin is much less certain. In people who have had their thyroid glands removed surgically, because of either a cancer, dangerously increased size (goiter), or excessive activity, there is no disease or syndrome that occurs as a result of lack of calcitonin hormone. There is no need to give replacement doses of this hormone to maintain good health. Calcitonin does not play a significant role in regulation of blood calcium levels. No bone loss pattern has been discovered as a result of loss of this hormone. In contrast, it is critical to replace the thyroid hormone that is lost after complete thyroid removal. (After partial removal, thyroid hormone replacement might not be necessary.)

During pregnancy and lactation, natural calcitonin levels increase. It is thought that perhaps calcitonin can help protect the mother's skeleton from the demands of the growing baby (both before and after birth). It is also possible that the existence of this hormone is obsolete—similar to what has happened with the appendix. It is still there because at one time it had an important purpose, but with evolution it has become unnecessary.

Calcitonin is digested and inactivated if taken orally (like insulin and PTH—see chapter 18) and thus not absorbed into the bloodstream or exposed to bone. Therefore, the only way to give the medication was at one time with an injection under the skin—not a deep muscular injection, but an injection nonetheless. When I first began working in the field of osteoporosis in 1988, the only medications available to treat or prevent the disease were estrogen or hormone regimens and injectable calcitonin. The medicine was given only once a day—a lot easier than insulin, for example, which is given multiple times each day.

In any case, in high doses it does have the ability to help preserve bone. This was first seen in laboratory studies using bone cells, where calcitonin could potently stop the bone-resorbing cell (the osteoclast) from doing its work and also stop bone loss in various animal models. There have been a fair number of relatively small randomized controlled trials evaluating the effect of injectable calcitonin on bone mass, and in general they suggest that bone loss of the spine or forearm can be arrested with this drug. There are no studies looking at injectable calcitonin's effects in the hip region. There has only been one small randomized clinical trial indicating that injectable calcitonin could reduce risk of vertebral fracture. No data have shown that calcitonin in any form can reduce the risk of hip fracture. Injectable calcitonin is almost never used anymore because we have better and more potent agents with fewer side effects that are easier to administer.

In any case, the injections turned out to be the easy part; the hard part was that patients often got very nauseated from this medication. I will never forget one of the first patients I admitted to my rehabilitation hospital—a woman in her sixties with rather severe osteoporosis who sustained a classic vertebral compression fracture from osteoporosis while trying to lift a stuck window. She was in severe pain, and I was advised to give her calcitonin by injection, which was thought to have pain-relieving properties. The practice, at that time, was to give a small test dose to make sure there was no allergic reaction. The patient became nauseated and vomited repeatedly for about twenty-four hours. I felt terrible—can you imagine going through severe back pain and then having it compounded with nausea and vomiting? That was one of my first and few experiences with that drug.

Fortunately, a unique form of the drug was introduced in 1995. The drug was administered via a nasal spray and approved by the FDA for the treatment (but not prevention) of osteoporosis. This method of delivery produces very few side effects, in contrast to the injectable variety, but it also seems to be a fairly weak agent in terms of its effectiveness on several of the intermediate outcomes (such as bone density) we typically measure in randomized clinical trials.

Intranasal calcitonin or Miacalcin (Novartis) was a big advance over injectable calcitonin when it was introduced in 1995. Several randomized controlled trials showed that it could prevent bone loss in women who were more than about five years beyond menopause. Women within five years of menopause are undergoing rapid bone loss from acute estrogen deficiency, and intranasal calcitonin is not potent enough to stop this loss. We participated in a multicenter trial evaluating intranasal calcitonin in women early after menopause; the results showed that calcitonin was not effective in this population, and we could never get the paper published. The FDA has the data, however, and it has been specific about not approving nasal calcitonin spray for prevention of osteoporosis (where many women in this early menopausal period would be treated) or for treatment in early postmenopausal women.

In women who are more than five years past menopause, when the dramatic menopause-related increase in bone turnover calms down a bit, nasal calcitonin spray can produce small increases in bone mass at the spine, but no increase in the hip region. The largest study employing nasal calcitonin and the only study for which we have fracture data for nasal calcitonin is called the PROOF study (Prevention of Recurrence of Osteoporotic Fractures). At the time this study was designed, it was groundbreaking. Remember that no medications other than estrogens and injectable calcitonin were approved for osteoporosis treatment at the time that nasal calcitonin was being developed and neither had large trials with fracture outcomes. A study of 1,255 people with osteoporosis sounded large and well designed. In fact, the initial size of the study was very reasonable for the outcome that was being assessed. The size of randomized controlled trials is always determined in advance by using estimates of the difference you expect to see between the control and active treatment groups and estimates of the frequency of the event you are looking for (powering the study). All the patients enrolled in this study were supposed to have vertebral fractures on their baseline set of spine X rays. It turned out that several hundred of the participants did not actually have evidence of vertebral fractures on their baseline X ray. As a result, fewer women were correctly enrolled in the study than expected.

A big limitation of this nasal calcitonin study is that there was a very large dropout rate during the investigation. Usually, 15 to 25 percent of patients withdraw from clinical trials in osteoporosis. In the PROOF study, 60 percent of patients dropped out before the investigation was finished. PROOF was planned as a five-year study; however, while the study was ongoing, the FDA approved the use of intranasal calcitonin for protection of bone density and treatment of osteoporosis in women who were more than five years past their last menstrual period. Since this was a placebo-controlled trial (25 percent of all participants were on placebo) and the study was blinded (neither the investigator nor the participant knew what dose of medicine the participant was on or if the participant was on a placebo), many patients opted to drop out of the study and actually take the medication once it came out on the market. Also, another more effective medication (alendronate; see the next chapter) also was approved by the FDA while the PROOF study was still in progress. Another group of women dropped out of the study to take this medicine. It is difficult for any volunteers to continue in a five-year placebo-controlled trial, but particularly for women who already have osteoporosis with established vertebral fractures. This is a long period for any woman to go without proven effective therapy. This might have made it difficult for investigators to urge patients to continue in the study.

Thus conclusions regarding the PROOF study are limited by the reduced number of women with appropriate entry criteria enrolled and the very high dropout rate. There were three different doses of calcitonin given. The approved dose is 200 IU. That dose produced a very small increase in bone mass at year one but thereafter, bone mass results were no different from the slight increases seen in the placebo group. The increases in placebo-treated women were unlikely to be real increases but were probably related to accumulation of calcium due to degenerative disease in the spine. This is very common in the spine as people age, and makes the spine's bone density sometimes less meaningful in older women than that of the hip. The results of this study also highlight the importance of looking at results in the medication group compared to the placebo group to guarantee that any changes seen are really from the medication rather than other factors (such as degenerative disease).

The changes in bone remodeling were similarly weak, with minimal differences compared to the placebo group. The vertebral fracture results were surprising because only the 200 IU dose of calcitonin produced any significant effect against fractures. The higher dose in the study did not produce any significant effect. Furthermore, the 200 IU dose had no effect on hip or any nonvertebral fractures.

THE BARE BONES

- Intranasal calcitonin is a medication with few side effects and no serious adverse effects.
- While it may have some effectiveness against vertebral fractures, calcitonin is probably the weakest of the approved medications and has no effect on fractures other than those of the spine. Therefore, it should only be used after trying other medications with greater proven effectiveness in older women with osteoporosis who are at risk for hip fracture.
- Calcitonin may have some pain-controlling effects, particularly on osteoporosis-related vertebral fractures.

Chapter 17

Bisphosphonates

CASE STUDIES

A sixty-nine-year-old previously healthy woman tripped over an irregularity in the sidewalk and broke her ankle. The fracture was serious enough that surgical pinning was required, and it took several months before she was walking normally again. Her doctor recommended a bone density test, which indicated that she had significant osteoporosis: Her T-Score was −2.8 in the spine and −3.2 in the hip. This patient is a good candidate for a once-weekly regimen of Fosamax to reduce risk of future fractures and treat her osteoporosis. Furthermore, her diet was low in calcium, so she should take a 600 mg calcium supplement with 200 IU of vitamin D, along with a daily multivitamin containing 400 IU of vitamin D and 200 mg of calcium. She should also be referred to a physical therapist to begin a muscle-strengthening program in addition to walking two miles three times a week.

A fifty-eight-year-old female bumped into a piece of furniture and broke a rib. A bone density test revealed a low hip

BMD T-score of –2.7, though her spine BMD was essentially normal at –1.4. She was a good candidate for Actonel 35 mg once weekly to treat her osteoporosis and reduce risk of further fractures. Since her diet already included milk, yogurt, and calcium-fortified juice daily, a calcium supplement was not necessary. She did, however, need to increase her activity level. She decided to join a gym and participate in a low-impact aerobics class twice a week, as well as Pilates once a week.

Bisphosphonate compounds have a long and interesting history. Closely related substances called pyrophosphates were originally used as detergents, as antiscaling agents to prevent deposition of calcium carbonate deposits in water pipes, and for other similar industrial indications. These pyrophosphates are still used in antitartar toothpastes and in nuclear medicine radiologic procedures such as bone scanning (not bone density testing).

Pyrophosphate compounds are also present in body fluids and probably act in some way to naturally regulate the amount of calcification in bone. Since these compounds are largely degraded when given orally, they have limited clinical applications. Similar compounds called bisphosphonates were subsequently developed for medical use, primarily by a physician-scientist named Herbert Fleisch.

At least five different drugs in this class are currently available in the United States for a variety of different bone diseases. They are subclassified by chemical structure, primarily by whether they contain nitrogen or not.

The bisphosphonate medications that are FDA-approved for the treatment of osteoporosis are:

- Alendronate (Fosamax, Merck)
- Risedronate (Actonel, Proctor and Gamble/Aventis)

A second subclass of agents that do not contain nitrogen and have lower potency than alendronate or risedronate includes:

- Etidronate (Didronel, Novartis) is used for Paget's disease and elevated blood calcium levels in certain cancers. It is also used in Canada and many European countries for osteoporosis, where it is usually given in a cyclic fashion, for two weeks every three months.
- Tiludronate (Skelid) is available in the United States and approved for Paget's disease.
- Clodronate is used both orally and intravenously. It is available in Canada and in many other countries (but not the United States) for tumor-related elevations in blood calcium and other cancer complications as well as Paget's disease.

A third subclass of bisphosphonate drugs has been developed primarily for intravenous use for treatment of cancer metastases to the bone and certain primary bone cancers, as well as elevated blood calcium levels. Since these medications avoid the gastrointestinal tract by avoiding oral administration, they may be an option for women who are unable to tolerate the oral agents:

- Pamidronate (Aredia)
- Zoledronic acid (Zometa)

There are data in the osteoporosis literature regarding these drugs. The former one, pamidronate, is not being developed for osteoporosis, but zoledronic acid is currently being evaluated in large osteoporosis treatment studies, the results of which should be available sometime near 2005. Since these agents are currently on the market for other specific conditions, they can be used for treatment of osteoporosis off-label. This is generally less desirable than using FDA-approved drugs but represents a potential alternative for people who really need bisphosphonate drugs and cannot tolerate the oral agents.

In this chapter, I'll try to briefly highlight the data for all the drugs available in the United States for osteoporosis. A few general principles are shared by all the medicines in this class. They are all poorly absorbed and must be taken on an empty stomach (see below for more detail). These medications may have some ability to limit the spread of cancer metastases, particularly to bone. They may accumulate in the skeleton and theoretically could have long-lasting effects months or even years after they are no longer taken. For the last reason, they do not have to be taken every day. Current treatments can be taken once a week; in the future, these medicines may exert effects for a whole year after a single intravenous injection.

ALENDRONATE

Alendronate is, at approved doses, the most potent oral bisphosphonate and probably the most potent of all of the antiresorptive osteoporosis medications currently on the market (distinct from PTH, an anabolic or bone-building medication, which will be discussed in the next chapter). Alendronate increases bone mass throughout the skeleton more than any other antiresorptive medicine and reduces bone turnover more potently than any other medicine. When it was first introduced, alendronate had to be taken every morning. The regimen was somewhat difficult because it had to be taken on an empty stomach with water only, and no other food or drink could be consumed for at least thirty minutes. More recently, alendronate was developed as a once-weekly agent. You need only take one pill (70 mg) once a week to get the same exact effect on bone mass and bone turnover as seen with a 10 mg pill every morning. This would be an advantage for many people with any medication, but particularly one whose regimen can be so demanding. If the medicine is taken with any drink other than water, however, or if there is any food in the stomach, its absorption is dramatically reduced and the described powerful effects will not be seen.

All of the results concerning alendronate come from extremely well-designed and well-performed randomized controlled trials. The largest study of the effectiveness of alendronate is the FIT or Fracture Intervention Trial. This was a two-part study: In the first part, called the vertebral fracture arm (which enrolled 2,047 women), all women had a vertebral fracture documented on X ray upon entry into the study, whereas in the second part, the clinical fracture arm (which enrolled 4,432 women), women were enrolled in the study by bone density definition of osteoporosis. Over half of the women were actually enrolled in the second part of the study in error. Their bone density T-Scores were originally calculated using the bone density measurement devices manufacturers' reference population. It turned out that this particular population was supernormal—their bone density values were actually higher than average for the young age group. As a result, the T-Scores of some of the patients entering this clinical trial appeared lower than they actually were when the T-Scores were recalculated using the much larger population from the National Health and Nutrition Education Survey (NHANES) involving more than 30,000 people. This is important for two reasons. First, it highlights the importance of using an appropriate reference population to calculate these T-Scores. Second, the population must be big enough and normal. Some of the new densitometry devices springing up do not have appropriate reference populations, and the resulting T-Scores are meaningless at best—or perhaps very misleading at worst. Another important point is that in people who do not have osteoporosis, it is difficult to show a protective effect against fractures, particularly those that occur in areas other than the spine.

Conclusions from the Fracture Intervention Trial in the women who did have osteoporosis are that alendronate reduced the risk of fractures of the spine by about 50 percent. Alendronate also reduced the risk of hip fractures and wrist fractures by about 50 percent. And it reduced the number of days of restricted activity or bed rest due to back pain, as well as disability days. From another study in women with osteoporosis that preceded FIT, alendronate actually reduced the amount of height loss over three years compared to women given placebo for the same amount of time. In fact, there are no other medications for which an ability to reduce height loss in the whole population has been shown. Finally, in another study among more than 1,900 women with low bone mass, alendronate reduced the occurrence of all nonspine fractures by about 50 percent. There are now also several meta-analyses (the highest level of medical evidence) in which the consistency of effects against vertebral and hip fractures has been shown.

Alendronate is FDA-approved for the treatment of osteoporosis related to long-term or high-dose steroid administration (see chapter 23) and also for the treatment of osteoporosis in men.

Side effects from alendronate are few. When it was first introduced, there were some cases where people were taking the medication without enough water and then lying down afterward. Without water to push the pill through the esophagus (the tube connecting the mouth to the stomach) into the stomach, and/or allowing gravity to aid in refluxing contents of the stomach (with the dissolved pill) back up into the esophagus, the medicine could produce irritation and sometimes even breakdown or ulceration of the esophagus. This was a recipe for disaster. A few people had serious problems. Since we learned how to administer the medicine, however, this has not been an issue. Some patients experience side effects such as heartburn or upper abdominal discomforts. Whether this is related to the natural ebbs and flows of underlying reflux disease or due to alendronate is unknown. Because reflux disease is so common and is seen with almost equal frequency in placebo- and drug-treatment groups in the alendronate studies, it is likely that this is largely related to the natural underlying situation. The clinical rule of thumb is to stop the alendronate if a person develops serious symptoms, let the symptoms subside—providing antacid agents if necessary—and then restart the alendronate a few weeks later. This almost always seems to work. If it doesn't, then another alternative medication should be tried.

The abdominal and gastrointestinal side effects of alendronate are reduced substantially when using the once-a-week regimen rather than the daily one. Some might think that taking a higher dose at one time might be detrimental, but in fact the likelihood of irritation is greater when taking the medicine more frequently. This is because the lining of the esophagus replaces itself every day or two, so that if there is any irritation then it is repaired and there is no further irritation for at least five subsequent days. One additional side effect that I have on occasion seen with alendronate is muscle and joint aches and pains. These are usually mild and go away after the person has been on the medication for a few weeks.

One of my favorite patients, who has severe osteoporosis, first came to my osteoporosis clinic with severe back pain due to multiple vertebral fractures that had all occurred within the preceding year. She had been started on a weak medication about six months earlier but had progressed with further pain and further compressions of the vertebral bones. After she had been on alendronate for about six months, the pain started to abate, and she has not had any fractures since. She often says that the treatment "saved her life."

RISEDRONATE

Risedronate is very similar to alendronate. It also produces potent effects on both bone mass and bone turnover. All the information we have on this drug comes from good randomized controlled trials. The first two studies showing fracture results using risedronate were all in women who had vertebral fractures at the time of entry into the study (called vertebral fracture studies or VERT). The two studies were identically designed, one performed in North America and the other in Europe; they enrolled a total of almost 3,700 women. Results indicated that risedronate could reduce occurrence of vertebral fractures by 40 to 50 percent over three years and could reduce all nonvertebral fractures by 33 to 40 percent.

These two vertebral fracture studies did not show any evidence that risedronate could reduce the occurrence of hip fracture, although a subsequent study specifically designed to evaluate the influence of risedronate on hip fracture occurrence did show effectiveness, at least in the group with the most severe documented osteoporosis. This was the largest osteoporosis study ever performed, called HIP, or Hip Intervention Program, and enrolled 9,331 women. There were two separate groups of patients: Group 1 included women between the ages of seventy and seventy-nine who had T-Scores lower than −3, while Group 2 included women over eighty who had a clinical risk factor for hip fracture, such as poor vision or previous falling. In the former group, risedronate reduced the risk of hip fracture by about 40 percent, whereas in the older Group 2, there was no significant reduction. The latter older group was unusual in that of the small percentage of women who actually had bone density measurements, only 16 percent had osteoporosis. This is far less than would be expected by age alone. Perhaps the explanation is that somehow volunteers in this age group were supernormal. The major message to learn from this is that bone density matters, even in the very old. In order to determine whether a medication for osteoporosis will work for a disease, it is important to first do the diagnostic test to show that the person has the disease.

I think that risedronate does probably work for hip, other nonvertebral, and vertebral fractures; still, the data are less consistent for hip fracture efficacy than they are regarding alendronate. The FDA has not yet allowed risedronate to be specifically indicated for prevention of hip fracture on the basis of the inconsistency in the study results. The side effect profile of risedronate is similar to that of alendronate. Risedronate has recently been approved as a once-weekly regimen similar to alendronate. There are no head-to-head comparisons of once-weekly alendronate treatment versus once-weekly risedronate treatment in terms of effectiveness or safety; one has recently been started. The weekly regimens of both drugs appear to have the same effectiveness as the daily treatments, and probably reduced side effects compared to daily treatments.

Risedronate is FDA-approved for prevention and treatment of osteoporosis related to high-dose or long-term steroid or glucocorticoid administration (see chapter 23). Although it does not have specific approval in men, it can be used for male osteoporosis.

ETIDRONATE

Etidronate is clearly weaker than the two agents that are FDA-approved for osteoporosis treatment, based on both in vitro and animal studies. The drug also has a potential side effect to impair the mineral content of bone. Bone is composed of a matrix of proteins and sugars, with calcium and phosphate mineral superimposed. Etidronate can impact the mineral content and thereby affect the quality of bone. Thus etidronate is usually given for two weeks out of every three months.

The quality of information that we have about etidronate in patients with osteoporosis is lower than that for alendronate or risedronate. There have been no very large studies evaluating the effectiveness of this drug for osteoporosis. None of the four studies done in women with osteoporosis has included more than 423 patients. Despite the small size of the investigations done with this medication, however, two of the four small studies showed a reduction in vertebral fracture in women treated with etidronate. None of these studies was big enough to evaluate fractures of sites other than the spine.

Although this agent may be an option for those who cannot tolerate alendronate or risedronate, the evidence base for effectiveness is lower, the potency of the agent is lower, and the possibility of interfering with bone mineral, especially after long-term use, is there. For all these reasons, it is preferable to use the approved agents when possible. Side effects of etidronate include diarrhea and abdominal pain. In contrast to alendronate and risedronate, etidronate can produce abnormalities in the amount of mineral deposited in bone and detrimentally affect bone strength if used in high doses for very long periods of time.

PAMIDRONATE

This agent has been around for longer than either of the bisphosphonates approved for osteoporosis. It has been used for treatment of bone cancer, elevated blood calcium levels associated with cancer, and Paget's disease of the bone. It has also been tried for osteoporosis in several clinical trials, of relatively short duration, with bone density improvement as the outcome but not reduced fractures. Bone density changes are consistent with what is often seen with bisphosphonates. In the studies, pamidronate was administered an average of every three months by intravenous (inside a vein) infusion. It must be administered over two to four hours each time. This agent remains an option for people who need treatment and who cannot take agents orally, but since there are no fracture data, the other agents should be tried first. Side effects can include fever and/or a flu-like syndrome the first day after the infusion. Muscle aches and pains can occur. Rarely, the arm through which the infusion was performed can develop irritation and/or infection.

ZOLEDRONIC ACID

This agent is approved by the FDA for the treatment of elevated blood calcium levels due to certain cancers. Recently, the agent was tested in a population of postmenopausal women in a variety of different dosing regimens. Results showed that after even a single infusion (over fifteen minutes) into the vein, the medication could reduce bone turnover for a whole year and improve bone mass to the same extent as administration of the same dose multiple times over the course of a year. There are as yet no fracture data with zoledronic acid; studies are currently being performed. This agent is very appealing as an osteoporosis therapy, but should only be used as a last resort at the current time since there is such a paucity of data. Ultimately, it may be possible to go to your doctor's office for a yearly checkup; depending on risk factors, including bone mass, the once-yearly osteoporosis treatment infusion could be given right at that time. There would be no issue of compliance with medication. Of course, patients would still have to be careful to ingest enough calcium, exercise regularly, and avoid detrimental habits, but this is still a lot easier than taking daily or weekly medication in addition. I think this medication, if it works the way we expect it to against fractures, will be an extremely compelling osteoporosis treatment.

DURATION OF THERAPY

It is unclear how long patients should stay on bisphosphonate medications. Since these agents are retained in the skeleton, it might make sense to stop at some point. If the agents are preserved intact in the skeleton, some might be released into the circulation by osteoclast degradation during the normal process of bone turnover and perhaps continue to work. The bisphosphonate could therefore serve as an ongoing depot of medicine. Another theoretical possibility is that there will be too much suppression of bone turnover. If this is the case, the bone will not be able to renew itself and it might ultimately fail as a result of impaired quality. Since there are not yet any very long-term data to evaluate this, we need to make reasonable decisions at the current time. My view is if patients are still in the osteoporosis range with regard to bone density, then the bisphosphonate should be continued. Among patients who have been on the drug already for four to five years, who have not had recent fractures, and whose bone density is above the osteoporosis level, it is reasonable to stop the medication at least for a year. Monitoring can be done with bone density testing and with blood and urine tests of bone turnover. If there is any sign of bone loss beginning, the medication can be restarted at that time.

THE BARE BONES

- Bisphosphonates are extremely strong agents for bone disease.
- Alendronate and risedronate improve bone mass, decrease bone turnover, and reduce the risk of fractures in the spine, hip, and elsewhere. These agents are the treatments of choice in older women (aged sixty-five-plus) with osteoporosis and also are very useful in younger women who do not wish to take either estrogens or raloxifene.
- In situations where alendronate or risedronate cannot be tolerated and very potent anti-osteoporosis agents are re-

quired, the off-label use of unapproved bisphosphonates can be considered.

- Zoledronic acid is currently being tested as a brief (fifteen-minute) infusion once a year for efficacy against hip and other fractures. Results should be available by around 2005 or 2006.
- The optimal duration of therapy with bisphosphonates is unknown.

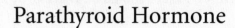

Chapter 18

Parathyroid Hormone

CASE STUDY

A seventy-year-old woman has had severe back pain for several months. When an X ray is taken, it is found that she has several compression fractures of the spine. Bone density testing confirms the diagnosis of osteoporosis. The spine BMD is not reliable due to fractures in that area, but the hip BMD T-Score is –3.

This woman is a good candidate for PTH treatment. She has severe osteoporosis and will benefit from a bone-building drug that will restore bone quantity and quality. After treatment with PTH for up to two years, a bisphosphonate medication should be started.

Parathyroid hormone (PTH) is one of my favorite subjects, since I have been working on the clinical utility of this medication for osteoporosis for about fourteen years. The first clinical research study that I ever participated in involved this compound. Although we have learned a tremendous amount about this compound during this time, there are still many unanswered questions. Certainly we can't assume that PTH is a cure for osteoporosis, but it is definitely a powerful medication that can reverse some of the structural as well as quantitative abnormalities associated with osteoporosis. It may work very well in combination with bisphosphonates or followed by bisphosphonates; studies ongoing right now are addressing these issues.

PTH is a naturally occurring hormone produced by the parathyroid glands—four small glands (hormone-producing organs) that sit adjacent to the thyroid gland at the base of the neck (thus giving them the name *parathyroid,* meaning "next to the thyroid"). Although these glands are in close proximity to the thyroid, they are in fact completely distinct functionally. They have nothing to do with thyroid hormone. If the thyroid is removed carefully, surgically, the parathyroid glands can usually be dissected off without causing any reduction in the function of the glands. PTH is the major calcium-regulating hormone of the body. When calcium levels in the blood go down during a period of calcium deficiency, PTH levels rise. PTH increases the absorption of calcium from the gut, helps retain more calcium instead of excreting it in the urine, and also increases bone breakdown, all in order to maintain normal blood calcium levels. The body will sacrifice bone, at least temporarily, to keep calcium levels within a very narrow range for optimal functioning of the nerves, muscles, heart—in fact all tissues of the body. In this setting, you might imagine that the PTH could actually be harmful to bone.

There are also conditions in which PTH is produced in excess by the body's own parathyroid gland, not in order to keep calcium levels up, but because of a benign tumor, for example. In this disorder, called primary hyperparathyroidism, the blood calcium levels might actually become elevated above the normal range. While this also can cause some bone dissolution and bone loss, particularly in the more severe forms of the disease, with mild disease there is usually no bone loss in the central skeleton of the spine, and often an actual higher level of bone mass can be seen there. This observation, showing that bone mass could actually be increased—in combination with a series of studies in animals given parathyroid extract dating back as far as 1929—stimulated interest in PTH as a therapeutic agent in the 1970s. It became possible to perform clinical studies in humans at that time, because the technology required to synthesize the hormone biochemically was developed. Prior to that, it was necessary to obtain PTH from animal sources by homogenizing their parathyroid glands.

Several studies performed in Europe, Canada, and the United States in the 1980s and 1990s showed that PTH could actually increase bone mass quite dramatically. When I give lectures to doctors on medication for osteoporosis, I am still frequently asked how this can possibly be good for the bone. As I mentioned above, we know of various conditions where it is clearly detrimental to bone. How could it ever possibly be helpful? This is still a very good question and a medical conundrum. We don't have all the answers, but we do know that PTH acts in a different way when it is given once a day than it does when elevated continuously in hyperparathyroidism or when it is elevated in response to low blood calcium. When we give it therapeutically for osteoporosis, the blood level of the PTH goes very high very fast and then comes back down to near normal. This seems to cause a different set of proteins to be made in the cells that manufacture bone, compared to the proteins made in the cells when PTH is always elevated. These proteins are associated with an increased ability of bone cells to produce more bone as well as a longer life span for each bone-forming cell.

The majority of controlled clinical trial data we have for PTH is in postmenopausal women, although there are two studies in men and one in premenopausal women with a disease called endometriosis. Endometriosis is a disorder in which uterine tissue grows outside the uterus into the pelvis and/or abdomen. It is often treated with agents that decrease estrogen production and can therefore cause bone loss. In one study, PTH prevented this bone loss. Studies in men will be discussed in chapter 21.

We can measure the effect of PTH to stimulate bone formation by levels of bone markers in the blood and urine. Both formation and resorption indicators are increased, but formation levels go up first. We also know that PTH can dramatically improve bone mass. It does this much more than increases from any of the other medical agents for osteoporosis; see figure 18-1. This can occur when the comparison group is placebo or when PTH is combined with another osteoporosis medicine such as estrogen or alendronate compared to that medicine alone. Recently, we learned that PTH can also increase the outer dimensions or diameter of bone. This is another mechanism by which it can improve bone strength. Lastly, we now know that PTH seems to be capable of actually restoring or improving the microarchitecture of bone. In osteoporosis, when you look at bone biopsy specimens microscopically, you usually see big holes in the tissue, similar to Swiss cheese. These big holes represent areas where cross-connecting pieces in bone have been dissolved. PTH can reconnect these pieces, and in effect might be able to completely reverse osteoporosis at least in certain parts of the skeleton (see figure 18-1). No other medications for osteoporosis can accomplish this. The other medications can help thicken some of the connecting struts inside bone, but they cannot reattach separated plates of bone to each other and actually fill in holes.

The largest clinical study of PTH treatment was a trial in

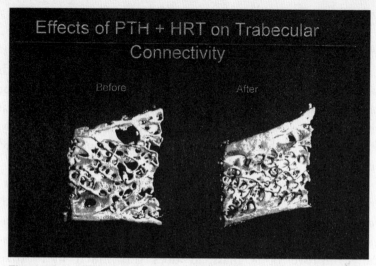

Figure 18-1: PTH not only increases bone density, but fortifies the inner structure of the bone itself. Reproduced from *J Bone Miner Res* 2001:1846–1853 with permission of the American Society for Bone and Mineral Research.

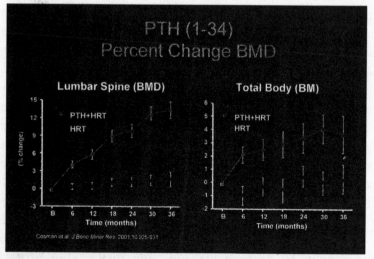

Figure 18-2: Studies have shown that PTH, in combination with HRT, can increase bone mineral density more quickly than can HRT alone. Reproduced from *J Bone Miner Res* 2001:925–931 with permission of the American Society for Bone and Mineral Research.

over 1,630 postmenopausal women with osteoporosis, all of whom had vertebral fractures on baseline X rays at study entry. The women were on no other medical treatment for osteoporosis except calcium and vitamin D. Two-thirds of the patients were assigned to different doses of PTH, and one-third were assigned to placebo. After approximately eighteen months of treatment, bone density of the lumbar spine in the approved-dose PTH group was 10 to 11 percent higher than placebo. Smaller differences in the hip and in total skeletal mineral content were seen between the PTH and placebo groups. Effects on the frequency of fractures were quite dramatic. There was a 65 percent reduction in the occurrence of vertebral fracture in the two PTH groups compared to the placebo group. With regard to nonvertebral fractures, PTH reduced the risk by between 45 and 55 percent, depending on the exact definitions used.

The fracture effects of PTH are dramatic, but perhaps *not so much greater* than fracture effects with either of the approved bisphosphonates—alendronate and risedronate. Since there are no head-to-head comparative studies big enough to address the potency of the two agents against each other, we can't be certain of the relative strengths of PTH versus bisphosphonates in the treatment of osteoporosis. More important than comparing these agents, though, is trying to understand how the drugs can be used together to reduce fractures. Toward this end, we know very little. The hope is that the effects of the bisphosphonates or other antiresorptive therapies (raloxifene, for example) could be used in combination with PTH. Since the drugs work by unique mechanisms, perhaps using the two drugs in sequence could provide an additive effect against fracture and truly approach a cure for osteoporosis. In fact, it will be recommended that an antiresorptive medication be started in almost all people after their PTH treatment to maintain all of the benefits.

SIDE EFFECTS

One of the biggest limitations of PTH is that it must be given by injection. The injection is into the subcutaneous fatty tissue (just under the skin), not a deep injection into the muscle. It is very similar to insulin injections in people with diabetes, but these must often be given multiple times each day. PTH is given once a day. I have enrolled in clinical trials patients well into their eighties who have not had difficulty giving themselves the medication, once they got used to the idea. Also, this is not an indefinite treatment: The course of PTH is generally not recommended to exceed twenty-four months.

Occasionally, blood and urine levels of calcium go above normal. This is more common with higher doses of PTH than it is with the approved dose. These levels usually return to normal spontaneously while treatment continues. Patients should not take excessive calcium while on PTH (or ever), but should continue to target recommendations of 1,200 to 1,500 mg per day (see chapter 6). Although a theoretical complication of having increased urine calcium is kidney stones, there were no increases in frequency of kidney stones in PTH-treated patients. Patients on PTH can have an increase in occurrence in leg cramps, nausea, headache, dizziness, joint pains, and general weakness, but all of these side effects are rare. Allergies and mild skin reactions at injection sites can also occur. A study in rats where PTH was given in high doses over the entire life span of the rat showed an increase in bone tumors. This finding is not thought to be relevant to humans.

FREQUENTLY ASKED QUESTIONS ABOUT PTH

Since PTH is such a new medication, there are many things we still do not know about the drug.

How long is the optimal course of therapy?

Probably between one and a half and two years. We know that with this treatment there are rapid changes in bone metabolism that can be measured in the blood and urine. Despite continuing the medication, these biochemical changes start to resolve, and within two to two and a half years they are not increased above baseline. Clearly, some resistance develops to this medication. We do not know why this happens, but it certainly seems to indicate that we should stop the medicine at this point. Bone mass might continue to go up even after discontinuing the PTH, because some of the bone tissue that was formed does not have its entire mineral content. When the mineral is deposited in normal concentration, it will be picked up in the bone density measurement.

Will it reduce hip fractures specifically?

We know that PTH has beneficial effects throughout the skeleton inducing reductions in fracture occurrence at the spine and all other sites after a year and a half. The largest study, though, was too small to evaluate the effectiveness of PTH on the hip per se. There were not enough hip fractures to know. In order to prove that PTH specifically reduces hip fracture risk, another larger clinical trial would have to be performed.

Can PTH be given a second or third time after an interval without PTH treatment and get a similar dramatic bone response?

This is an intriguing question. Right now, we know that PTH is very powerful on bone, improving both mass and architecture. However, for those women who start out with very low bone mass or who have had multiple fractures, the usual response to PTH will likely not be enough to restore them to a state where they have normal bone. These individuals might be helped by receiving another round of PTH for one and a half to two years. At this point, it is completely unknown whether a second course of medicine could actually work at all or as well as the first course of PTH. It is an area of active investigation at the moment.

Will the bone changes after PTH be retained after the medication is discontinued?

There is limited information on this issue. Still, from an investigation in men and from observations made from follow-up in the largest trial so far in women, it appears that bone will probably be lost in people who have had PTH-induced bone gains in the absence of an antiresorptive medication afterward. Most likely, in the absence of further medication, within a few years bone mass (and presumably architecture) will return to its pre-PTH state. Thus, PTH cannot be considered the only answer for treatment of significant osteoporosis. It can, however, restore bone to a much healthier state, in which an agent which prevents further loss is all that is necessary.

Should a bisphosphonate, raloxifene, or estrogen be given with PTH, after PTH, or before PTH for the best effect?

Nobody knows. If you put together all that is known so far, it appears that it probably doesn't matter what order the medications are given in. You seem to get an additive effect from the antiresorptive medication and the PTH whether the antiresorptive medication precedes, accompanies, or chases the PTH treatment. Ongoing investigations are studying this question currently. It may be that some combinations might produce better results than others, but it will take at least a few years to figure this out. At this moment, it looks like the most rational regimen would be PTH followed by a bisphosphonate.

Who should get PTH and who should not?

Practically speaking, it is likely that many patients who have mild to moderate osteoporosis by bone density definition should be started first on an effective antiresorptive medication. Those patients who still have osteoporosis by bone density after one to three years of this medication might benefit from a course of PTH. Those patients who have had significant osteoporosis-related fractures should probably also get a course of PTH. For those women who have had fractures or who have very low bone mass and have not been treated with a prior medication, PTH can be given alone for a course of about one and a half to two years. Based on the available data, antiresorptive medications should be started once the PTH course is finished.

The question of who should *not* get PTH is easier to answer. Women who have modestly or moderately low bone mass (above the osteoporosis range), without any prior adulthood or minimally traumatic fractures, should not get PTH. These people do not have bone mass disturbances low enough to justify use of PTH; nor are they likely to have bone structural disturbances serious enough to justify its use. People with Paget's disease, hyperparathyroidism, elevated blood calcium, or metastatic disease from any cancer should not receive PTH. People who have had radiation therapy to the skeleton and young people with growing bones should not receive Forteo. Furthermore, it may be prudent to avoid use in individuals recently diagnosed with cancers that can spread to bone, such as breast or prostate.

Will there be alternative forms of PTH available in the near future?

Obviously, taking medication by injection is less desirable than other ways of administering it. Because PTH is a small protein hormone, like insulin and calcitonin, if given by mouth it would be readily dissolved and digested in the stomach and intestine and be unable to retain its activity. Alternative delivery systems of PTH have been explored. These include a skin patch, an inhaler, and a nasal spray. So far, these have all failed for different reasons. Another possibility is that an oral formulation will be developed that can bypass the stomach and avoid digestion. While it is likely that alternative forms of PTH delivery will at some time be available, I think this is at least five years down the line (second half of this decade).

THE BARE BONES

- PTH is the only bone-building drug approved by the FDA for use in osteoporosis.
- PTH produces major beneficial effects on bone density but also increases bone size and quality. All of these effects contribute to substantial increases in bone strength and ability to resist breakage.
- While it may be possible to give PTH in combination with other osteoporosis medications, the sequence of treatment and the optimal duration of antiresorptive medication before, during, and after PTH are all unknown. Right now, I would at least recommend a bisphosphonate after PTH treatment.
- PTH must be given by subcutaneous injection (under the skin), similar to an insulin injection.
- PTH is most appropriate for people with moderately severe or severe osteoporosis.

Chapter 19

Non-FDA-Approved Treatments

ANABOLIC STEROIDS (ANDROGENIC STEROIDS)

The anabolic steroids, mostly synthetic derivatives of the male hormone testosterone, influence many body systems, including muscle, blood, and bone. They are considered investigational and are not approved by the Food and Drug Administration for use in osteoporosis.

Anabolic steroids appear to stimulate bone formation in women. In postmenopausal osteoporotic women with compression fractures, double-blind controlled studies of anabolic steroids such as stanozolol and nandrolone decanoate have demonstrated improvement in spinal, wrist, and total skeletal bone mass over two-year periods. Androgens might also have a positive effect on bone mass of the spine and hip when combined with estrogens. No studies, however, have shown a reduction in the occurrence of fractures with anabolic steroid treatment. Some small clinical trials indicate that low doses of testosterone might improve libido.

Levels of DHEA, an adrenal steroid, decrease dramatically

with age, and there is some suggestion—though it is not consistent—that levels might correlate with BMD. However, there are no convincing clinical trials to date indicating that DHEA administration can improve skeletal status.

Furthermore, the anabolic steroids have significant systemic side effects, including liver abnormalities, sodium and fluid retention, and masculinizing effects, such as hair growth, acne, and deepening of the voice. When administered continuously for extended periods in excess of those doses originally tested for osteoporosis, anabolic steroids can cause liver tumors. Lastly, anabolic steroids can adversely affect serum lipids, reducing the high-density lipoproteins and elevating the low-density lipoproteins, with a deleterious effect on atherosclerosis and coronary artery disease. Compounds that retain some of the benefits of anabolic steroids but avoid the other detrimental effects such as masculinization would be the best option for this class of drug, but such compounds have not yet been developed for clinical use.

Testosterone therapy is clearly indicated in men with deficiency of the hormone who already have osteoporosis or who are at high risk for developing it.

CALCITRIOL

Vitamin D (calciferol) is an essential sterol, synthesized in the skin following exposure to ultraviolet light (sunlight). In addition, vitamin D is available through the diet (fatty fish, eggs, liver, butter, and vitamin-D-fortified foods such as milk), or through multivitamin supplements. Vitamin D undergoes transformation in the liver to calcifediol (25-hydroxyvitamin D) and further transformation in the kidney to calcitriol (1,25-dihydroxyvitamin D). Calcitriol is the most potent vitamin D compound, although other forms may have some biological activity.

Published studies have shown inconsistent effects of treatment with active vitamin D (calcitriol) in increasing bone mineral density or reducing fractures. Furthermore, the therapeutic index is low such that doses of calcitriol that could perhaps result in a benefit to the skeleton may be very similar to the doses that result in excess urine and blood calcium levels. The use of the parent vitamin D compound (calciferol) in moderate doses is much safer. (See chapter 6).

FLUORIDE

Although fluoride has been used for approximately thirty years by a number of clinicians for the treatment of spinal osteoporosis, it remains an experimental therapy, not approved currently in any form by the FDA for such treatment.

Fluoride has usually been administered as plain sodium fluoride, but other forms have also been tested, including enteric coated tablets, slow-release forms, and monofluorophosphate. Fluoride produces a linear increase in spinal bone mass of 5 to 10 percent per year for up to four years in most (but not all) subjects and can also increase bone mass in the hip region. The marked increase in bone mass is a result of a stimulation of bone formation through an increase in the number and function of osteoblasts, the cells that make bone. The major side effects of sodium fluoride administration include gastrointestinal irritation, lower-extremity pain, and stress fractures. The gastrointestinal symptoms and, perhaps, the lower-extremity pain may be decreased with the use of enteric coated or slow-release forms of the drugs.

Several rigorous controlled trials of the use of fluoride in spinal osteoporosis have been published. One randomized multicenter trial (which was not placebo-controlled) showed that the proportion of patients with new vertebral fractures was significantly reduced at twenty-four months of treatment compared to patients receiving other forms of therapy. Two double-blind placebo-controlled trials (with a total of almost three hundred patients) of sodium fluoride at an average daily dose of 75 mg per day showed highly significant increases in spinal bone mass. However, no significant reduction in vertebral fracture rates was seen. Of more concern, there was a significant increase in peripheral fractures when both complete and stress fractures were included, possibly related to the toxicity of sodium fluoride at the dosage used. A reanalysis of a subset of the patients who had less dramatic increments in bone mass change showed a reduction in vertebral fracture incidence in this subgroup. Several recent European trials have shown conflicting results regarding effects against vertebral fracture using different forms of fluoride.

Recently, results of a randomized placebo-controlled trial of a novel form of the medication, slow-release sodium fluoride, were published. The study recruited 110 postmenopausal osteoporotic women and tested slow-release sodium fluoride at 50 mg per day for twelve of every fourteen months for four and a half years. Ninety-nine women remained in the study for more than one year and were analyzed. Women in the fluoride arm had a significantly lower vertebral fracture rate (57 versus 85 percent).

Currently, sodium fluoride, in all of its forms, must continue to be considered experimental, and patients should only use this agent in clinical trials.

GROWTH HORMONE AGENTS

In people who are truly growth hormone deficient, growth hormone and its analogues might improve bone mass. There is also a decline in production and secretion of growth hormone with aging. It has therefore been postulated that growth hormone agents might be useful in the treatment of osteoporosis. Several small studies indicate that growth-hormone-type agents can stimulate the bone remodeling process, although the bone mass increments seen with these therapies are very modest and not consistent with a true bone-building effect on the skeleton.

In contrast, short-term trials of growth-hormone-type medications do show an increase in lean body mass and reduction in fat mass. Small increments in BMD might be occurring as a result of the changes in body composition rather than as a direct effect on BMD. The change in lean body mass may be itself very important, however. There are no medications right now that can reliably and safely improve lean body mass. Improvements in lean body mass might be expected to reduce frailty in older individuals; improve strength, coordination, and balance; and possibly reduce the frequency of falls in the elderly. This could have a dramatic effect on reducing the risk of important fractures, particularly those of the hip. Growth hormone itself must be administered by injection because it is a small protein hormone, like parathyroid hormone and insulin. Side effects include fluid retention and sometimes the development of carpal tunnel syndrome as well as joint pains, muscle pains, and local skin reactions at injection sites.

Analogues of the growth-hormone-releasing factor are currently under investigation. These agents stimulate the body's own production of growth hormone, and some can be given orally. These drugs have potential therapeutic value, not so much for their bone effects as for their other effects on body composition.

NITRATES

These medications, used for many years for people with heart disease—particularly angina symptoms—may have some protective benefits to bone. There is some preliminary evidence indicating that they have mild antiresorptive and perhaps even mild bone-building properties. If these preliminary data are confirmed, nitrates could be an effective and relatively inexpensive way to help treat osteoporosis. It will take over five years before we will know.

STATINS

These agents are truly miraculous medications for elevated blood cholesterol. They are highly effective at reducing serum cholesterol levels, reducing fatty plaques in arteries, and reducing the risk of heart and other vascular diseases. In the process of inhibiting steps in the cholesterol synthesis pathway, they also reduce the quantities of several compounds that affect functioning of both osteoblasts and osteoclasts. Studies in cell cultures as well as animal models reveal that statins can stimulate bone formation and also reduce bone resorption. Potentially, these two mechanisms could result in a substantial improvement in skeletal mass and architecture.

There are also a number of observational cohorts indicating that statin use is associated with a dramatic reduction in the risk of fracture, particularly hip fracture. Not all studies are consistent with these findings, however. The early short-term prospective data in humans, including some from our group, have so far shown no consistent stimulation of bone formation when these agents are administered orally. It may be that concentrations of the agent are too small in bone when administered by mouth, where the medication is metabolized in high concentration at the liver. Some preliminary data looking at a transdermal (through-the-skin) preparation in animals indicates that the agents might have a greater effect when administered in this form. Larger longer-term investigations concerning various statin compounds have been recently started. At this time, the statin drugs still hold some promise as bone-active agents, but it would be unwise to assume that statin users are protected from or adequately treated for osteoporosis.

STRONTIUM RANELATE

Strontium is a heavy metal that has been studied almost solely in Europe for more than ten years as a treatment for osteoporosis. It is said to possess both antiresorptive effects (like most of the medications currently marketed) and anabolic activity (like PTH). Both of these effects are modest in magnitude. The metal is incorporated into bone and raises bone density, in part as an artifact of its presence in bone, and in part perhaps because of its actions on bone metabolism. Results of a multicenter clinical trial indicate that strontium might in fact increase bone strength and produce some protective effect against vertebral fracture occurrence at three years; nonvertebral fracture data have not been analyzed, however, as of the writing of this book. It is unlikely that strontium will be approved in the United States in the near future.

THIAZIDES

Thiazides are actually diuretic agents (stimulating the excretion of excess fluid) used primarily to treat high blood pressure, fluid retention, and sometimes heart failure. Thiazides can actually reduce urine calcium excretion and possibly improve calcium balance. Several observational studies indicate that thiazide users have a reduced risk of hip fracture and a higher bone mineral density. These findings could be explained by the increased weight often found in women who have high blood pressure. Two small randomized controlled trials in older women showed modest benefits on bone mass of about 1 percent over two to three years versus control groups. Although it is possible that thiazides could have an adjunctive role in the prevention or treatment of osteoporosis, it is premature to recommend these agents for the general population at the current time.

There are some women and men who excrete too much calcium in the urine. Although all of us lose some calcium through our urine, some of us excrete calcium in excess. This can put our calcium balance in jeopardy. This is a problem that should be considered in all young people with osteoporosis-related fractures or very significant osteoporosis. Also, those who have had kidney stones should be tested, since high urine calcium can be a cause of both osteoporosis and kidney stones. Many of these individuals would benefit from treatment with a thiazide, which can reduce the risk of both diseases.

TIBOLONE

Tibolone is a synthetic agent that has some estrogen-type effects, some progestinlike effects, and some testosteronelike effects. It is approved in countries other than the United States for menopausal symptoms. It produces these disparate effects in part because it is metabolized (converted) to different agents in the body. It seems to decrease hot flashes and night sweats, as estrogens do. It also produces modest increases in bone mass in postmenopausal women, but we have no data on its ability to reduce occurrence of fractures. In the breast, its effects are distinct from those of estrogen. It does not increase the density of breast tissue (a risk factor for breast cancer) the way estrogens do. Whether it can reduce the risk of breast cancer or simply produces no effect is uncertain at this time. In the uterus, tibolone might have neutral effects, but its long-term safety on the uterine lining is still to be determined. Preliminary data show that it can have some benefits to cholesterol levels, but the ultimate effects on the heart are unknown.

THE BARE BONES

- None of the medications or substances discussed in this chapter has enough solid evidence to recommend that patients take it for treatment or prevention of osteoporosis at this time.
- Women who are interested in finding out more about osteoporosis and/or contributing to medical knowledge and the development of more effective therapies for osteoporosis should consider entering a clinical trial.
- Some of the agents discussed in this chapter are being tested in clinical trials currently, and others are on the horizon.

Chapter 20

Monitoring Treatment

It is difficult to imagine that people would be willing to take a medication for many years to prevent consequences from a disease that produces no symptoms in its early stages in the absence of any objective evidence that the medication is working. The analogy would be to expect people to continue antihypertensive medication without measuring blood pressure or to continue statin or other cholesterol-lowering drugs without ever measuring cholesterol levels. It is imperative, therefore, that we have some objective monitoring tools to determine that a treatment is working and to help convince people to stay the course with lifestyle changes and medication. The occurrence of fractures is not adequate for monitoring since fractures are generally not that frequent in one individual. Therefore, the lack of fractures over a one- or two-year period is not terribly reassuring. Similarly, the occurrence of an osteoporosis-related fracture in an individual does not mean that a treatment has failed. We can never know that more fractures would not have occurred in the absence of treatment.

Height measurements can be a good indication of progression or halting of progression of osteoporosis of the spine. People who sustain vertebral compression fractures usually lose height; however, such loss of height is not totally specific to osteoporosis, so that we should not assume that spinal fractures have occurred in those with height loss. Reductions in height can be related to degeneration of the cartilage-containing disks between the vertebral bones, which happens with age to some extent in almost everyone and can produce up to two inches or sometimes even more loss in height. In those people who have scoliosis—a worsening of the sideways curvature of the spine totally distinct from complications of osteoporosis—height loss often occurs.

In a person who has known osteoporosis and prospectively measured height loss, an X ray of the spine should be performed to determine if new or worsening compression fractures have occurred. At this time, the X ray is the definitive diagnostic tool to answer this question; however, it is possible and may be standard to obtain this information from bone densitometry equipment in the future.

The only tools we have right now for osteoporosis treatment monitoring are height measurements, bone density measurements, and measurements of biochemical turnover indices in blood or urine. Neither bone density testing nor biochemical measurements in blood or urine is a perfect monitoring tool. In the case of the bone density measurement, only small changes are expected with the majority of our current medicines over one to two years. These expected changes may not exceed the precision error of the measurement. In other words, as in all analytical methods, there is inherent error in the determination itself even if the variation in the body is expected to be extremely small (no day-to-day variation in bone density). The best monitoring tool would produce a large expected change with medicine compared to a small precision error. Often when it comes to bone density readings, it is unclear if the change seen is actually real or just related to analytical error.

The same is true for the biochemical markers. Although rather large changes in these blood and urine test levels are expected after initiating treatment of osteoporosis, there is also a large variability in levels even from day to day in individuals. Therefore, this is not a perfect test either, with consistent reductions of 30 to 50 percent usually required on a follow-up level compared to the baseline level to be sure that there is a true medication effect. While this is often seen with the strongest medications—alendronate and risedronate as well as estrogen—it may not always be seen with raloxifene or calcitonin. Monitoring with these latter agents is probably best done with bone density testing.

One of the advantages to using biochemical marker tests for monitoring is that changes are possible to appreciate at an earlier time point than those seen with repeat bone density measurements. For example, it would not make sense in almost any circumstance to repeat bone densities before at least one year of therapy. In contrast, the biochemical tests usually show an effect within about three to six months of treatment.

In my clinical practice, I often obtain a test of bone turnover prior to starting therapy. The one I believe is the most clinically valuable at the moment is the urine or serum n-telopeptide or NTX test. This test can sometimes be used for risk assessment (as discussed in chapter 11), to help decide if treatment is needed when bone density and clinical risk factors are inconclusive. In this case, though, I'm recommending using it for purposes of monitoring; a baseline level prior to starting treatment is the optimal way to do this. After treatment has been initiated, a repeat urine determination is performed, usually within about six months. If the original level, prior to treatment, is actually low (indicating low bone turnover at baseline), then it might not be helpful to repeat the test. If the original level was high, however, then a repeat determination that shows the level to be substantially reduced can be reassuring that the treatment is probably having the desired effect. There are no data right now confirming that this type of approach actually improves the adherence to a medical program, but it certainly might in individual cases. Of course, the biggest determinant of how adherent a person is to a specific medical treatment is probably how effective the doctor is in explaining the need for the medicine and actually sitting down and talking to the patient about the whole disease process. Spending time with patients tends to motivate people to at least try what is being recommended.

I always repeat bone density measurements on people in whom I initiate medical therapy. The average time is about one year after starting treatment, although an argument can be rationally made to wait for two years. With the most potent medicines, waiting two years means that there is a great likelihood of seeing an increase in bone density that can be considered truly significant. We have to be very careful interpreting the measurement, though, primarily since treatment changes should not generally be based on the follow-up measurement, even if a bone density increase is not seen, particularly in women who are already on the most potent therapies. Sometimes it is likely that an individual who does not gain bone but instead remains stable might have actually lost a substantial amount of bone during the follow-up period had she not been started on treatment. Also, until end of November 2002, there was little to offer a woman already on potent osteoporosis treatment and not gaining bone. Now that PTH (Forteo) is approved for treatment, this might represent an option for people who are not increasing on bisphosphonates and still have very reduced bone mass. Once it is clear that the medication is being taken correctly and regularly, in most individuals the best thing to do is wait for another bone density test the next year. Here the urine n-telopeptide test can also be helpful. If the bone density is not increasing as expected, at least if the urine NTX level is reduced (with bisphosphonate treatment) it can reassure both the patient and doctor that everything is probably fine.

One last comment about serial bone density assessments: There is a phenomenon called regression to the mean, which applies here. This is a mathematical concept that also applies to some biological conditions. Individual patient results tend to get closer to the mean or average response as time goes on. So, for example, if a woman has bone loss despite being treated with alendronate in the first year, chances are she'll have a big positive response the second year. The opposite is also true: Women who have a big increase in the first year often have a small decrease in the second. This is another reason that you don't want to be too quick to abandon a therapy.

THE BARE BONES

- We don't have perfect monitoring tools for osteoporosis therapy.
- An accurate measurement of height is clearly important, especially for people who have osteoporosis of the spine.
- Repeat X rays are appropriate for some people who have had vertebral fractures or deformities or who experience back pain, changes in back or trunk shape, or height loss.

- If you are about to start treatment for osteoporosis, ask your doctor if a bone turnover marker such as a urine or serum NTX or serum CTX should be obtained. It can then be repeated within six to twelve months of starting treatment.
- Repeat bone density measurements can be performed after one to two years of therapy for monitoring of treatment effect.
- Patients and doctors must be careful when interpreting the results of both biochemical markers and bone density results for monitoring. There is inherent variability in both these measurements, and it's wise to be very sure that the follow-up results are really very disparate from expected results before changing medication, particularly when one of the more potent medications is being used.

Part V

SPECIAL CASES

Chapter 21

Men

Osteoporosis is more common in women than in men, but it is still an extremely common condition in men. For example, the lifetime risk of a hip fracture in men is about 6 percent (six in one hundred men will have one), whereas the lifetime risk for a woman is about 15 to 17 percent. At the age of fifty, the likelihood of having osteoporosis by BMD measurement of hip, spine, or wrist is about 35 percent in women and about 19 percent in men. Approximately one in four Caucasian men will suffer an osteoporosis-related fracture at some point in his lifetime. This is a greater lifetime risk than that of developing prostate cancer. Also, men tend to have greater problems than women after suffering certain fractures, particularly those of the hip, and are at greater risk for dying in the year following the hip fracture than are women. The likelihood that a man will return to the fully independent lifestyle he had prior to the hip fracture is even lower than it is for a woman. When men require stays in rehabilitation hospitals after a hip fracture, they usually stay longer than women.

Many of the risk factors for women are the same for men,

such as family history of osteoporosis, personal history of fracture, having a small frame or low body weight, taking medications such as steroids, or having certain underlying endocrine or rheumatologic diseases. Some of these diseases include AIDS, chronic lung disease such as emphysema or chronic bronchitis, Type I diabetes (insulin requiring), hyperparathyroidism, inflammatory bowel disease, chronic kidney or liver disease, rheumatoid arthritis, malabsorption problems including gastric or duodenal surgery, and neurologic diseases such as Parkinson's disease or multiple sclerosis. Men also have increased risk if they make too little testosterone—similar to the phenomenon of menopause in women, when estrogen production dramatically declines. Heavy alcohol ingestion or alcoholism and smoking are also important risk factors for osteoporosis in men. In men with prostate cancer, use of gonadotropin-releasing hormone analogues such as lupron can increase the risk of bone loss and osteoporosis. Excessive use of thyroid hormone or lack of monitoring of thyroid hormone therapy as well as chronic need for blood-thinning medications, chemotherapy or immunosuppressive drugs for certain rheumatologic diseases, or organ transplants also increase the risk of bone loss.

Besides the presence of osteoporosis, the other major determinant of fracture risk in men is falling (just as it is in women). Falls can be related to frailty or specific medical problems, including low body weight or weight loss, poor nutrition including deficient protein intake, chronic diseases, low physical activity, muscle weakness or neurologic diseases (Parkinson's disease is a common one), problems with cognitive functioning, and the use of sleeping or anxiety medications or other medicines that can cause sedation.

The prevention of osteoporosis in men is similar to that in

women. Any possible risk factors should be eliminated or reduced. Major attempts at smoking cessation should be made. Alcohol ingestion should not be excessive, and alcohol abuse should be specifically treated. Calcium intake should be maintained at about 1,000 to 1,200 mg per day in younger men and at least 1,200 mg per day in men fifty and older. Similarly to women, vitamin D intake should be between 400 and 800 IU per day, depending on age. All men should engage in regular physical activity, preferably weight bearing (standing on your feet) and muscle strengthening of the large muscle groups—back, shoulder, hip, and pelvic muscles.

Those men at high risk should strongly consider a bone density test. Currently, there are no well-accepted guidelines as to which men should undergo this test. These are being developed and will likely come out of a large epidemiologic study called "Mr. Os" over the next few years. This study will look at both the frequency of fracture occurrence and its relationship to bone density as well as the importance of other risk factors, such as family history. It will provide us with the age at which osteoporosis risk is high enough that routine testing should be recommended. This will probably be between age seventy and seventy-five. Obtaining reimbursement for bone density testing from insurance companies will probably follow from the guidelines expected in the next several years.

The actual values on bone density tests in men come out higher than those in women since men on average have a higher BMD than women. This may in part be due to genetically predetermined gender difference and in part be related to the differences in body size, weight, and bone size. The gender difference is probably not there at birth but develops during puberty, when boys gain substantially more bone than girls, in part related to gaining more height and bone length at this stage of life. When you look at smaller men and compare them to larger women, you see less of a gender difference in bone density. In fact, bone size alone is a mechanically protective factor against osteoporosis for men. Larger bones are more resistant to mechanical stresses than smaller bones, so larger men have generally lower risk than smaller women.

Nevertheless, on average men have bone densities about 5 to 10 percent higher than those of age-matched women. Currently, the most accepted way of defining osteoporosis in men is by calculating T-Scores in much the same way we do for women. Thus, an individual man's bone density values are compared to those of young healthy men, and the difference between the average young man's and the patient's score is calculated as standard deviation scores just as for women. A T-Score of −2.5 or below in a man is in the osteoporosis category, just as it would be in a woman.

Bone density testing is presently indicated and definitely reimbursable for the following conditions: men found to have a vertebral compression fracture or thinned bone on X ray; men who have been treated with steroid medications such as prednisone for three to six months or more; men with a diagnosis of hyperparathyroidism; and men being treated for osteoporosis. I would also advocate bone density testing in men who have had substantial height loss (one and a half to two or more inches), more than one adulthood fracture in the absence of significant trauma, and men with any of the conditions mentioned above. Check with your insurance company to find out if it will cover the cost of the test.

Men who do have vertebral fractures on X ray do not always have osteoporosis, however. It is believed that because men have in general more active lifestyles than women, some of the deformities that show up on X ray are actually traumatic and not related to osteoporosis. While this may be true of some women also, it is more common in men.

If you have been diagnosed with osteoporosis, you should make sure you are getting at least 1,200 mg of calcium each day (through the diet and a supplement if necessary). You should get between 400 and 800 IU of vitamin D per day. Make sure you are engaging in physical activity, preferably weight bearing and muscle strengthening through a resistance program. Measures to limit the risk of falling should be instituted. There are also medical treatment options. Alendronate and PTH (Forteo) are both approved by the FDA for the treatment of osteoporosis in men, but risedronate is also an option. Studies of alendronate and PTH in men are much smaller than those in women and only efficacy against vertebral fractures has been shown (as well as increases in BMD).

In short, we have less information at this time about osteoporosis in men because most of the initial research was performed in women. Since the disease is far more common in women than men, this approach made sense, but current research efforts are aimed at making up for this inequity. If you are or know a man who has osteoporosis or is worried about it, follow the advice outlined in part II of the book and consult a doctor about whether testing or treatment is recommended.

THE BARE BONES

- Men have higher bone mass than women because of bigger body and bone size as well as other genetic factors.
- Men do not have accelerated bone loss in midlife, as do women at menopause, but men do experience ongoing age-related bone loss just like women.

- Men have a lower osteoporosis-related fracture risk than women—but it is still substantial. Approximately one in every four white men will have one of these fractures.
- Men have a worse prognosis after hip fracture than women.
- Risk factors for men are similar to those for women and include personal fracture history, family history of osteoporosis or fractures, smoking, alcohol abuse, and many chronic diseases and medications.
- Men should follow the preventive measures outlined in this book, including getting enough calcium and vitamin D, exercising regularly, and avoiding smoking and excessive alcohol consumption.
- There are two medications approved for the treatment of osteoporosis in men: alendronate (Fosamax) and PTH (Teriparatide or Forteo).

Chapter 22

The Premenopausal Woman

Women who have not had a menstrual period in a year or more are considered to have gone through menopause. Women who are still having regular periods are considered premenopausal, and women who are having irregular periods, particularly in their late forties or early fifties, are considered to be in the perimenopausal period of life.

As I discussed in the beginning of this book, I do not advocate routine bone density testing of premenopausal women at the current time. There are no medications proven safe or effective yet in this age group, and many women are inappropriately started on medication or are excessively worried about having a reduced bone mass or osteoporosis. All premenopausal women should follow the bone health program outlined in part II of this book: Maintain a healthy calcium- and vitamin-D-enriched diet or supplement if necessary, engage in regular weight-bearing and muscle-strengthening exercise (at least three times a week), don't start smoking or quit if you are currently smoking, and don't drink excessively.

There are times, however, where bone density testing is

necessary or may be recommended in premenopausal women. Some of these cases are in young women who have had multiple prior fractures in the absence of major trauma. For example, premenopausal women who have had spine, rib, or other fractures in falls or other minor accidents should have bone density testing. Certain osteoporosis conditions manifest themselves in young people, and in these cases where serious fractures have already occurred, if osteoporosis is confirmed by bone density testing then medication might be warranted, even in the absence of good evidence supporting effectiveness and safety. It is my opinion that these women should only be treated by specialists in the field of osteoporosis or endocrinology, who are most likely to make the appropriate decisions about initiating, monitoring, and ultimately discontinuing medications.

There is a specific entity called transient osteoporosis of pregnancy. In this form of osteoporosis, previously healthy young women can actually have spine or hip fractures during the third trimester of pregnancy or within a few months after delivery of the baby. It is a very rare condition—almost always occurring with a first pregnancy—and one into which we have little insight. It is not clear why women get this and how to avoid it. As the name implies, osteoporosis associated with pregnancy usually goes away within a few months of the baby's birth. If a bone density test is low at the time of pregnancy when the fracture occurred, when it is repeated a year or two later the bone density may be normal. Thus the person usually does not suffer from chronic osteoporosis. In fact, most of the cases that have been reported in the medical literature suggest that the condition will not recur in future pregnancies. In general, since the condition is transient and the age group being considered is still in the childbearing range, it is usually not necessary or recommended to begin medication. On the other hand, in young women who do not improve their bone mass but instead remain in the osteoporosis range, especially those who are done with childbearing, medication could be considered. As in the situation above, I believe this should be done only in consultation with a specialist.

Certain diseases that often begin during the premenopausal phase of life have detrimental effects on the skeleton. One of the most important of these conditions is anorexia nervosa. In this very serious eating disorder, osteoporosis is due both to the self-imposed starvation—with its accompanying loss of nutrients needed for regrowth of bone tissue—as well as to the dramatic weight loss, usually accompanied by loss of estrogen production and menstrual periods. Although osteoporosis can be severe and is one of the most important complications of anorexia nervosa, the only way to treat the osteoporosis is by treating the underlying condition. Treatment of anorexia often requires a multifaceted approach involving psychiatrists for medication recommendations, psychologists or other counselors, nutritionists, general physicians, family, and community support programs. There is no way to correct the osteoporosis without alleviating the primary disease. Oral contraceptive pills to initiate menstrual periods and provide estrogen to the skeleton might be useful while the disease is being treated, but if it is treated effectively, the return of body weight and body composition is usually associated with a return of menstrual function. Supply of adequate calcium and vitamin D is important in addition to calorie and protein replacement.

If left untreated or not treated effectively, anorexia nervosa is often terminal, and osteoporosis is the least of the person's problems. In people who recover from anorexia, some but probably not all of the bone mass deficit is reversible. If a young woman recovers from anorexia and now eats normally, has a normal weight and normal menstrual cycle, but still has osteoporosis, a specific osteoporosis treatment is usually not indicated. Certainly in women approaching or just past menopause who have had anorexia nervosa in the past, early bone density testing should be performed. Treatment is often required at that stage to prevent any further skeletal deterioration.

In contrast to anorexia nervosa, the other major eating disorder, bulimia, with repeated binging and purging, is not characteristically associated with osteoporosis. Eating disorders may be mixed, however, with anorexic phases still putting young women at risk for osteoporosis.

Excessive exercise can also produce abnormal menstrual function, particularly at levels sometimes required for elite athletics and elite dance. Such extreme physical training is often associated with abnormally low body weight and sometimes anorexia. The whole combination of disorders is sometimes called the female triad—the combination of anorexia, excessive exercise, and lack of menstruation. Women with the female triad condition need to reduce their physical training, eat more and with better concentration on optimal nutrition, and allow menses to return to normal. The short-term rewards of being extremely competitive in sports or dance must be balanced by the long-term detriments to physical and perhaps psychological health.

There are other conditions that can cause low estrogen levels and affect menstrual function in young women. All may be associated with bone loss, and bone density testing may be recommended. One of these conditions is attributable to treatment of endometriosis (where the lining of the uterus extends outside the uterus into the abdomen or elsewhere). In this condition, menstrual periods can be very painful, and infertility may result. The treatment sometimes involves a medication that can decrease estrogen levels. Some chronic illnesses, such as kidney or liver disease, are associated with weight loss and bone loss. Abnormal thyroid hormone production (excess or deficient) can cause abnormal menstrual function. Certain pituitary gland or hypothalamus tumors can produce hormone excesses or deficiencies, producing abnormalities in menstrual function. Lastly, sometimes estrogen deficiency ceases as a result of ovary disease per se, a condition usually causing menopause at the average age of fifty or fifty-one. When occurring before age forty-five, it is considered premature ovarian failure, and may co-occur with other autoimmune diseases. Abnormal menstrual function as a result of any of these conditions should prompt treatment of the underlying disease; osteoporosis treatment should be considered only after the disease has been treated. Low bone mass can be a result of abnormal growth hormone levels or treatment of a seizure disorder. For all of these conditions, the disease should be treated first. Generally, specific treatment for the osteoporosis per se is not required.

A large group of diseases that can and do often begin during young adulthood can be associated with osteoporosis. The diseases include: Type I diabetes, AIDS, hyperparathyroidism (excess parathyroid hormone, causing calcium levels to rise in the blood), hyperthyroidism (excess thyroid hormone), ulcerative colitis and Crohn's disease, chronic kidney and liver disease, lupus, celiac disease (also called gluten-sensitive enteropathy) or other illnesses causing malabsorption, and neurologic diseases such as multiple sclerosis, rheumatoid arthritis, and scleroderma. It is good to be aware that these diseases can contribute to osteoporosis risk. It may make younger women more apt to follow bone health measures. The presence of these conditions should also alert women to ask for bone density testing at or near the time of menopause. In general, bone density testing is not advocated, however, during the pre-menopausal period, even in people who have these conditions, since treatment options have not been evaluated in these groups. Still, in younger women with chronic disease who have had fractures, the benefits of bone density testing and treatment might outweigh any possible risks.

THE BARE BONES

- If you are a healthy premenopausal woman, follow the bone health steps discussed throughout this book: Make sure your calcium intake is adequate and that you get some vitamin D, get regular weight-bearing aerobic and muscle-strengthening exercise and maintain good posture during all activities, don't smoke, and don't drink excessively. At the time that menstrual periods become irregular or infrequent, review your risk factors for osteoporosis and ask your doctor then to refer you for a bone density test.
- If you have had a vertebral or hip fracture during premenopausal adulthood that occurred with little trauma, ask your doctor to refer you to a specialist in osteoporosis.
- If you have had a fracture that occurred with minimal trauma during a pregnancy, ask for a referral to a specialist to consider the diagnosis of transient osteoporosis of pregnancy.
- If you have had multiple fractures with little trauma during your adulthood, ask your doctor to refer you for a bone

density test. If the results are in or near the osteoporosis range, ask for a referral to a specialist in osteoporosis.

- If you are about to initiate steroid treatment for a proposed period of more than a month, ask your doctor to refer you for a bone density test.

- If you have a serious chronic illness, such as kidney or liver disease, rheumatoid arthritis or lupus—particularly if you have had a fracture that occurred with little trauma—ask your doctor if a bone density test should be done.

- If you are having very infrequent menstrual periods or long times without a menstrual period, see your doctor to determine and treat the cause. If the periods never return, ask for a bone density test.

Chapter 23

Osteoporosis Associated with Steroids

All people who require long-term or high doses of steroids—also called glucocorticoids or corticosteroids, and including prednisone and cortisone—are at risk for bone loss. Bone loss is probably the most serious side effect of steroid treatment. Steroid treatment is used for a variety of autoimmune or connective tissue diseases, including rheumatoid arthritis, ulcerative colitis, Crohn's disease, lupus, and asthma. Obviously, patients should be on the lowest possible dose of steroid for the shortest possible period of time. It may, however, be impossible to limit steroid exposure to an amount that is not detrimental to bone.

Steroid-induced bone loss may occur at low doses and may be extremely rapid, particularly in those bones containing large amounts of cancellous or porous bone, such as the vertebrae of the spine. Oral steroid treatment might lead to losses of 5 to 8 percent of bone mass in the spine in the first five or six months of therapy. Steroid inhalers and steroids that are injected into the joint are less damaging to the skeleton than orally administered forms but can still produce dose-dependent adverse effects.

Steroids upset the balance between bone dissolution (resorption) and bone formation such that more bone is broken down than formed under the influence of these drugs. Within hours of receiving high-dose steroid medication, bone formation is shut down. Furthermore, steroids are linked to the death of a type of bone cell called the osteocyte, which is responsible for helping repair damaged bone. With decreased numbers of osteocytes, bone quality might be impaired. Steroids are associated with a reduction in the efficiency of calcium absorption from the intestine and an increase in calcium excretion in the urine. Therefore, steroids can affect both the quantity (bone mass) and the quality of bone as well as interfering with calcium balance and affecting calcium supply.

It has been shown recently that steroids result in a very high rate of osteoporosis-related fracture while they are being administered. A large British trial evaluated 244,235 adults from England who had received oral steroids and compared them to an equal number of individuals matched for medical practice, age, and gender who did not receive any oral steroids. Fracture occurrence was directly related to steroid use and dose. In those people who received daily doses of 7.5 mg or more of the commonly prescribed prednisone (or its equivalent), the risk of having a vertebral fracture was more than five times greater than among people not receiving steroids. Also, the risk of hip fracture was more than two times greater in steroid users than nonusers. Even in those people receiving lower doses of steroid (between 2.5 and 7.5 mg per day) there was an increase in the risk of fracture of the spine (almost threefold) and of the hip (almost twofold).

Another equally important discovery from this study was

that the elevated fracture risk associated with beginning and continuing steroids began almost immediately after initiating the steroid treatment. Similarly, the fracture risk returned to rates seen in non-steroid-treated individuals rapidly when the steroids were discontinued. These observations indicate that any treatment that is going to be optimally effective for prevention of osteoporosis should probably be initiated before starting steroids and continued while steroids are being used. It may very well be possible, though, that osteoporosis medications started in this manner can also be stopped if the steroid treatment can be stopped. Other observational studies and controlled intervention trials indicate that age, gender, and menopausal status affect fracture risk in individuals on steroids. Several of the controlled trials show that premenopausal women on steroids do not suffer from vertebral fractures over a one- to two-year follow-up period. Fractures in men were intermediate between the essentially zero fractures in premenopausal women and the high number seen in postmenopausal women. Moreover, many of the factors that contribute to increased fracture risk in normal healthy postmenopausal women also contribute to the risk of osteoporosis in steroid-treated women—age, family history, and so forth.

The diagnosis of steroid-induced osteoporosis is the same as in normal primary osteoporosis (osteoporosis where there is no specific underlying disease or medication responsible). A bone density test must be done to determine baseline risk at the time steroids are to be administered. The decision to treat with an effective medication must be made in light of the person's BMD result, age, and other associated risk factors, including the severity of underlying disease and the likelihood of requirement for chronic steroid treatment.

Although not everyone about to embark on a course of steroid treatment requires medical therapy, preventive measures should be followed in everyone. These are the same universal measures that should be followed by anyone interested in bone health, steroids or not. Any accompanying risk factors such as smoking or alcohol abuse should be treated. When possible, doses of steroids should be reduced and inhalers used in place of systemic steroids. Measures to help reduce the risk of falls should be instituted. Exercise is essential both for its effects on reducing bone loss and for its muscle-strengthening effects, which might help maintain lean body mass and agility, reducing the risk of falls. Furthermore, individuals with steroid-induced osteoporosis should optimize nutrition. Calcium and vitamin D may be effective at reducing bone loss during chronic steroid administration, although they are not sufficient at preventing bone loss in those about to start steroid treatment. It is recommended that all people on steroids consume at least 1,200 mg a day of calcium (or up to 1,500 mg) and up to 800 IU per day of vitamin D.

While hormone replacement therapy is often recommended for glucocorticoid-induced osteoporosis (GCIOP), only one randomized, very small, controlled trial of HRT in women on steroid treatment has been performed. That study showed a modest increase in spine BMD but no statistically significant effect on hip BMD and was far too small to evaluate fracture outcome. A few small investigations of injectable and nasal calcitonin indicated some preservation of spinal BMD but no effect on hip BMD and no vertebral or other fracture data.

By far the most convincing studies for GCIOP are those in which bisphosphonates were utilized. Both alendronate and risedronate are FDA-approved for GCIOP treatment, and risedronate is also approved for GCIOP prevention. Alendronate was tested in a one-year trial with a one-year extension in 477 patients either on established chronic steroid therapy or about to begin treatment. The study included men, postmenopausal women, and premenopausal women. BMD in the spine increased 3 to 4 percent over the first year compared to the placebo group. There was a further increase in BMD in the second year. Smaller but significant increases in hip BMD were also seen. Fractures did not occur in the premenopausal women, but in postmenopausal women the number of X-ray-diagnosed vertebral fractures was substantially reduced in those taking alendronate.

Risedronate was tested in 224 patients about to begin steroid treatment. It had beneficial effects on both spine and hip BMD and substantial effects on vertebral fracture occurrence. Also, in a treatment study of patients who had been on steroids chronically, BMD increased throughout the skeleton. Risedronate produced a dramatic reduction in vertebral fracture occurrence over the course of this trial. Etidronate also appears to have some efficacy in GCIOP but is not FDA-approved for this indication. PTH has also been studied in patients with GCIOP and looks effective for people with this disorder.

At this time, it is prudent for all postmenopausal women and adult men about to begin glucocorticoid treatment to have a bone density test. If the BMD results are in the range of -1.5 or below, medical therapy with bisphosphonates should be considered. The treatment does not need to be continued beyond the course of steroids. Once steroids are stopped, the bisphosphonate treatment can usually be stopped. In premenopausal women who are still in the childbearing years, treatment can be considered; however, it should be stopped if an incipient pregnancy is possible. The ultimate safety of bis-phosphonate treatment on future pregnancy has not been established. All patients who have already been on long-term steroid treatment should be offered a bone density test, and treatment should be offered to those with osteoporosis or significantly reduced bone mass.

Despite intensive development efforts to identify other medications with fewer detrimental side effects, steroids remain the treatment of choice for many autoimmune conditions. At least we now have medication that is highly effective at mitigating the skeletal toxicity associated with their use.

THE BARE BONES

- Steroids are extremely effective at treating a variety of chronic diseases but result in bone loss and a high rate of osteoporosis-related fractures during their use.
- If you are about to begin steroids for a proposed period of more than one month, you should request a bone density test. If your bone density level is in the range of −1.5 or below, treatment with a bisphosphonate would probably be recommended.
- If you have already been on steroids for a prolonged period (three months or more), you should request a bone density test. If bone density is close to −2 or below, treatment with a bisphosphonate would probably be recommended.
- If you are about to begin or have already been treated with steroids, make sure you are getting at least 1,200 mg of calcium in your diet (or diet plus supplements) each day and at least 400 to 800 IU of vitamin D each day. You should engage in regular exercise (ideally weight-bearing and

muscle-strengthening exercise, but modified according to the limits of the underlying disease for which the steroids are being taken). You should quit smoking and avoid excessive drinking.

Afterword: The Future

The future of research and treatment of osteoporosis looks bright from here. Improvements in methodology for diagnosis and treatment are guaranteed. Some of these new techniques include:

- We will probably abandon the whole T-Score system and base everything on five- to ten-year absolute fracture risk assessments: The bone densitometry equipment will calculate risk based on gender and age. Then the absolute risk will be modified by weight and other clinical risk factors (fracture history, family history, and so forth).
- We will have new guidelines in which we recommend bone density testing for all women at menopause and for all men at a certain age, perhaps by age seventy.
- Diagnosis of abnormal vertebrae using DXA will become standard. X rays will not be required to diagnose vertebral fracture.
- We will have ways to noninvasively measure bone microarchitecture and quality.

- We will have agents besides PTH that can rebuild bone and help people who have established osteoporosis or severely reduced bone mass.
- We will have drugs that can be administered very infrequently (such as the once-yearly zoledronic acid) or will be even more powerful than those we have now.
- We may have ways of genetically manipulating the skeleton, perhaps an ability to infuse a high-bone-mass gene and dramatically improve bone mass.
- We may have medications that can augment muscle mass, improve strength, and increase coordination, thereby reducing frailty and falling.
- We will determine exactly which exercises can exert the most dramatic effects on the skeleton.

Incorporating these progressive methods with the augmented data we'll receive from studies currently under way, doctors and patients will be better informed and equipped to prevent, treat, and help reverse the punishing effects of osteoporosis.

As I mentioned at the beginning of this book, the current state of the U.S. medical system simply doesn't allow time for doctors to comprehensively explain all the inner workings of such a complicated condition as osteoporosis. For this reason, I hope that this book has filled in some of that gap to empower you with the tools you need to prevent disease and engage in a proactive discussion with your doctors. I hope that what I've learned in my fifteen years of experience taking care of patients with osteoporosis empowers you and your skeleton to live a long, healthy, strong life.

Interpreting Medical Evidence

It is important if you are going to be a wary consumer to understand how we determine what modalities are truly effective in preventing or treating osteoporosis. This appendix will help you separate the noise from the news. Here, I'll discuss the types of evidence that are available when looking at a product's effect on osteoporosis. This approach is valid for products marketed for other diseases also. It will discuss no specific compounds, but provide a general description of the hierarchy of medical evidence, from the personal testimonial, to the laboratory, to animal models of disease, to observational studies in humans, to the most convincing forms of medical evidence—the randomized controlled clinical trial and the summary of clinical trial evidence called the meta-analysis.

PERSONAL TESTIMONIALS

The lay literature is replete with misinformation, most of which is related to herbal or other nutritional remedies. Many people seem to believe or want to believe advertising about these remedies and probably think that because these substances are called supplements or vitamins, for example, and not drugs, they certainly are safe. I believe that all the substances you ingest in pill form are drugs or medications. To me, it makes no sense to take any of these medications unless there is proof that they work. Nutritional supplements are not subject to the same standards for approval and marketing as medications, and therefore the companies that make these compounds often do not spend the money or time to try to prove that they work. I have also found it interesting over the years of seeing postmenopausal women with various issues how easy people find it to criticize the pharmaceutical industry: "They're all in it just for the money." Well, what do they think the CEOs of the nutritional supplement companies are in it for? For some reason, people find it easier to believe that the latter companies are not interested in financial profits. This is a very shortsighted view of industry in general.

Since the companies that make nutritional supplements are not well regulated with respect to their health claims, for many of these products there is no more evidence than personal testimonials suggesting that they may be helpful. Personal testimonials are simply statements from one or more individuals making a claim, such as: "I used BoneSuppXXX and I felt strong and had no fractures." First of all, many people—even those with severe osteoporosis—can go months to years without any fractures. In this example, there is no duration of use or follow-up period of time. Second, feeling strong has nothing to do with most agents used for bone disease. Feeling strong is more likely related to how much sleep you have had in the last week, how much exercise you've been getting, how regular your eating habits have been, and what your overall mental/emotional state is. Third, any individual can feel any way with or without a substance. The so-called placebo or sugar pill effect is a very powerful one. If people think they will feel a certain way, then a large percentage of the time, they do feel that way. In other words, from a few individuals' statements, we certainly could not conclude that BoneSuppXXX is going to treat, prevent, or cure osteoporosis. Despite this, many people buy BoneSuppXXX. Furthermore, because BoneSuppXXX is a nutritional supplement rather than a drug, people assume that it is safe, without side effects. There are no drugs or nutritional products without side effects.

Personal testimonials are the lowest level of medical evidence; they really have no predictive value whatsoever for determining the effectiveness of a medication. It is mandatory to have a control group when we want to study the effectiveness of a medication. In contrast to the language of the personal testimonial, the kind of language that a pharmaceutical product could use after performing controlled clinical trials is: "Our drug was tested in a study of three thousand people who all had osteoporosis. Half of the group was assigned to receive our medication and half of the group received a placebo pill. Over three years of follow-up study, the people assigned to the medication group had an improvement in their bone density and a reduction in both spine and other fractures. There was less height loss in the medication-treated group and less back pain. Our drug was associated with only a slight increase in risk of headache." This is the kind of evidence that could convince me to recommend a product——supplement or drug.

LABORATORY STUDIES

Laboratory studies are almost always done at the beginning of any drug evaluation. These are studies of the drug's effect on pertinent cells or organ culture systems in the laboratory. This is the first way to test whether the drug might have the desired effect on the target tissues, but it is obviously a long way from this stage to proving that a drug works in humans. This now mandatory stage in drug testing helps supply the underlying biology or physical process that suggests a drug might work for a certain disease. Laboratory testing has become so sophisticated that we now can actually determine what genes are being activated and what proteins are being made when we administer drugs to cell systems. Molecular biology and proteomics are two totally novel branches of science that have developed and blossomed only over the last ten years. Knowing that Drug X works for osteoporosis and does so by increasing transcription of Gene A and translation to Protein B might allow us to develop another drug, an even more potent or ultimately safer, more tolerable compound. Designing drugs targeted to have specific effects on production of important proteins beneficial to bone health, rather than trying compounds off the shelf to see if they work, is where the field of osteoporosis will be moving in the next decade.

ANIMAL MODELS OF DISEASE AND DRUG EFFECTS

Studies in laboratory animals are the next level of evidence supporting the effectiveness of a drug. These are often performed first in rodents, rats, or mice, and then usually in another mammal, such as a rabbit. While the concept of using animals for experimentation is abhorrent to many of us, it is a good way to try to determine both efficacy and, just as importantly, safety before giving the medication to humans. Obviously, like most of you, I support the idea of treating animals with complete humanity, and not performing unnecessary experiments. However, all drugs being evaluated by the FDA for ultimate approval to treat a certain disease require animal models of drug efficacy and safety. These studies require meeting institutional standards for animal care and use, which assures that humane standards are met. Studies of the influence of medication on animal models of disease help supply the biologic rationale (in addition to the in vitro cellular studies above) to help support the concept that a drug might be effective. Animal studies have become increasingly sophisticated, as indicated above with respect to laboratory studies. Once we suspect that a certain gene may be involved in a disease process or drug effect, we can genetically breed a mouse to have this gene removed (the knock-out mouse) or amplified (born with extra copies of the gene). We can then determine the exact importance of that gene in disease and treatment.

OBSERVATIONAL STUDIES

Studies in humans are the last form of medical evidence, but there are several levels of human research that need to be considered. Human investigation can be broadly classified in two categories: observational study and randomized clinical trial. Observational studies include retrospective and prospective types. In the retrospective study, people who have had a problem such as a hip fracture are identified (cases). They are compared with a group of people of similar age who have not had a hip fracture (controls). Both groups are then asked a series of questions, such as: Did you smoke and for how long? Did you ever take estrogen? At what age was your menopause? How much milk did you drink when you were a child? How much alcohol did you drink as a young adult? We then compare the proportion of cases with a particular response in the hip fracture group to the proportion of cases with the same response in the control group. For example, if 90 percent of the time people who have had a hip fracture have a history of never drinking milk, in contrast to 10 percent of the time that people who have not had a hip fracture drank no milk, we might be able to make the association between never drinking milk and having a hip fracture.

Perhaps when reading through these questions, you noticed that it might be difficult to answer some of them. This is one of the biggest problems with these case–control retrospective studies. They force people to try to remember many things from the distant past, and there may be many inaccuracies associated with this. The accuracy of the conclusions that are drawn from this type of observational study depends obviously on the accuracy of people's memories. In addition, people who have already had a hip fracture might answer questions differently.

It is also important to realize that these studies allow us to determine possible associations between certain factors and the development of hip fracture, but they may not allow us to determine specific cause and effect. For example, we cannot be sure that a lack of milk consumption resulted in an increased risk of hip fracture rather than that lack of milk consumption may be due to an intestinal disease, or perhaps even that lack of milk consumption may be a marker of lack of exercise, or smoking, or drinking too much soda, or following a generally poor diet. Thus, the hip fractures might actually have nothing to do with the lack of milk consumption.

Another form of observational study is called the prospective cohort study. In this type of study design, we identify a large group of individuals of a certain age and get a lot of information about them. We may get historical information again, similar to that mentioned above. Then people in the study are followed for a period of time—five to ten or more years. During this time, they are monitored for the development of the disease about which the study is most interested, in this case hip fracture. This type of study allows us to also take blood, urine, and various X-ray imaging tests before the hip fracture occurs to determine their predictive value with regard to the likelihood of having a hip fracture. Furthermore, information about diet and other lifestyle habits, the influences of other diseases, and many other factors can be gleaned from this kind of study. Also, it relies less on memory and more on the factors that may be pertinent at the time that the study started.

The observational studies in general are not applicable to looking at the effectiveness of medications, because in general—and certainly in the current era—medications must pass much more vigorous tests to get on the market. In the past, however, medications could get on the market more easily. We then could observe the long-term ramifications in people who used the medications. Also, sometimes an observational study could help us determine that a drug approved for use for disease X might seem to have an effect also on disease Y.

Of the two basic types of observational studies, the prospective cohort study has much more power to ferret out important things than the case–control study and we can be sure that the risk factor preceded the hip fracture. However, both observational studies are critical for generating hypotheses. They allow us to hypothesize, for example, that estrogen use might be important in preventing hip fracture. Importantly, though, in general these studies are not definitive. It is almost impossible to control for all the things that may be associated with, for example, the selection of estrogen use in a prospective cohort study. Estrogen use may be associated with a greater education, better nutrition, more exercise, better overall health, less smoking, and many other factors, some of which may not even be known. This potential problem of additional factors that may go along with the one being analyzed in this type of investigation is called bias. With respect to estrogen use, it is called healthy cohort bias. Some things—such as how one disease affects another—can only be evaluated in an observational study. One example is the influence of rheumatoid arthritis on osteoporosis.

RANDOMIZED CONTROLLED TRIALS

Many of the hypotheses that are formulated in observational investigations can be subsequently tested in more definitive studies called randomized controlled trials. These trials provide the highest level of medical evidence available. Randomized trials are currently the industry standard for proving that a drug really works and are required by the FDA before a drug can be approved for any indication. In these studies, a group of individuals are identified. They are then randomly assigned, usually with the help of a computer, to receive a medication or placebo—a sugar pill designed to look just like the medicine. Usually in these studies, neither the investigative team nor the individual who is in the research study knows whether the person is on the active drug or the placebo. They are all "blinded" to treatment assignment. This helps prevent any subjective influences regarding belief in the drug from affecting the results of the study. The randomization is the most important element of these definitive studies. This assures (if the study is large enough) that the people who get into the active treatment group will be similar to the people who get into the placebo group. Therefore, there should be no equivalent to the healthy cohort bias in this kind of study. The two groups should be very similar except for the one intervention that the study is based on.

There are two basic types of randomized controlled trials in the field of osteoporosis. They involve the intermediate outcomes (such as bone density and biochemical tests of bone turnover) and the ultimate disease outcome (fracture occurrence). While we must first prove that a medication works on the intermediate outcome, ultimately for a drug to be shown as an effective agent for osteoporosis treatment, we must also prove that it works in preventing fractures in good randomized clinical trials. It generally takes a much bigger and/or longer study to show an effect against fracture occurrence rather than on bone density. In part, the number of patients required to prove efficacy against fracture outcome is related to the likelihood of the event occurring. Women who have already had fractures have a much higher risk of future fractures, so that the most efficient way to design a study looking at the effectiveness of a drug for osteoporosis is to choose this high-risk group. Women who have osteoporosis by bone density testing but have not yet had fractures are the group at second highest risk. The size and importance of a study also depends on the specific fracture outcome. For example, many more vertebral or spine fractures occur in people with osteoporosis than hip fractures. Furthermore, it may be that certain medications can work on one type of fracture and not on another. Specific examples of this difference are discussed in the specific treatment chapters of this book.

Generally, when we think about medications for prevention of osteoporosis, we only require that bone density remain stable rather than expecting a decreased risk of fracture. The likelihood of fracture occurrence over a few-year period of time in women who do not yet have osteoporosis is too low to assess unless the study is enormous in size—perhaps about the size of the WHI (16,000 women) for five years, instead of two to ten thousand patients who have osteoporosis already for three years (depending on specifically which fractures you are looking for). It is hoped and expected that preventing bone loss in women who do not yet have osteoporosis will ultimately be reflected in a long-term reduction in the risk of fractures. In the optimal world, we would have long-term studies with fracture outcomes for drugs approved for osteoporosis prevention; in the real world, however, the cost would be extremely high, and it might be difficult to retain patients on a placebo for such a long period of time.

All randomized placebo-controlled trials include a control group that does not take any active medications, except usually calcium and sometimes vitamin D. While it may seem unethical that some women could be on an ineffective medication, medical science could not progress without these courageous individuals. Nor would we ever really have the answer about whether a drug works. An institutional review board for human subject research reviews all trials before they can be performed, and every individual must sign an informed consent. The risks and benefits of participation in the study are detailed. Any person can withdraw from participation in a research study at any time. Moreover, there are specific caveats usually written into research protocols such that patients will be taken out of the study if (for example) they lose a lot of bone.

Lastly, those women at extremely high risk of having a fracture would not be good candidates for randomized controlled trials.

META-ANALYSES

Most people consider the meta-analysis of randomized controlled trials to be the strongest form of evidence available to evaluate a drug. These meta-analyses search the medical literature for all of the controlled trials evaluating a specific drug. The authors make sure that there are no serious flaws with any of the studies. Then they pool all of the data and get an average summary of the effects. This type of analysis allows you to determine how studies with slightly different results can be viewed. When the meta-analysis is done well, it can be extremely helpful. Sometimes, however, the conclusions are not stronger from a meta-analysis than they are from one large, really well-performed randomized controlled trial.

THE BARE BONES

- It is important to be critical about personal-testimonial advertisements for compounds. First, many might not even be true, but second, without a control group and a sufficient sample of patients, it is impossible to know if the claim is due to the treatment or just a change in the person's condition or perception.
- When treatments are being tested for osteoporosis, they first have to undergo laboratory testing, then testing in animals, and finally in humans.
- It is possible to be misled about the effects of certain medicines when conclusions have come only from observational studies. One example is the effect of hormone replacement on heart disease (see chapter 14).
- The effectiveness and safety of medications, supplements, and other treatments for osteoporosis—as well as other

conditions—should be tested in randomized controlled trials, the highest level of medical evidence.

- For a treatment to be proven effective in osteoporosis, the drug has to reduce the risk of fractures in patients with osteoporosis. For a medication to be approved for osteoporosis prevention, it has to prevent bone loss and reduce bone turnover.

Web Sites with Good Information about Osteoporosis

GENERAL INFORMATION ABOUT OSTEOPOROSIS

National Osteoporosis Foundation
   http://www.nof.org
New York State Osteoporosis Prevention & Education Program
   http://www.nysopep.org
Osteoporosis and Related Bone Diseases National Resource Center
   http://www.osteo.org
National Osteoporosis Society
   http://www.nos.org.uk
International Osteoporosis Foundation
   http://www.osteofound.org
Foundation for Osteoporosis Research and Education
   http://www.fore.org
Osteoporosis Patient Resources
   http://www.imaginis.net/osteoporosis
Strong Women, Strong Bones
   http:/www.strongwomen.com
Local Osteoporosis Education Link
   http://www.LOEL.net

INFORMATION ABOUT EXERCISE FOR OSTEOPOROSIS

Sara Meeks Physical Therapy
   http://www.sarameekspt.com
Mirabai Holland
   http://www.mirabaiHolland.com

INFORMATION ABOUT MENOPAUSE

National Institute on Aging
   http://www.nia.nih.gov
North American Menopause Society
   http://www.menopause.org

NUTRITION INFORMATION

The American Dietetic Association
   http://www.eatright.org
Food and Nutrition Information Center
   http://www.nalusda.gov/fnic.html
National Institutes of Health
   http://www.nih.gov

MEDICATION INFORMATION

Food and Drug Administration
   http://vm.cfsan.fda.gov/~foodlab.htm

DIETARY SUPPLEMENT INFORMATION

NIH Center for Complementary and Alternative Medicine
    http://altmed.od.nih.gov

INFORMATION ABOUT FALL PREVENTION

Centers for Disease Control and Prevention
    http://www.cdc.gov
Hip Protectors
    http://www.hiprotector.com
Safehip
    http://www.safehip.com

WEB SITES FOR KIDS AND TEENS

Powerful Bones. Powerful Girls. The National Bone Health Campaign
    http://www.cdc.gov/powerfulbones
Bone Builders: An Osteoporosis Awareness Campaign
    http://www.bonebuilders.org
Bone Health Education Website
    http://kidshealth.org/kid/grownup/conditions

WEB SITES FOR SPECIAL POPULATIONS

Celiac Sprue Association
    http://www.csaceliacs.org
Celiac Disease Foundation
    http://www.celiac.org
Gluten Intolerance Group of North America
    http://www.gluten.net

Index

Page numbers of illustrations appear in italics.

Actonel (risedronate), xii, 193, 207–9,
　259–60
age
　bone density tests and, 104–6
　bone loss and, 121–22
　bone strength and, 31
　bone turnover and, 27, 133
　osteopenia and, 122
　osteoporosis and, 25, 104–6, 121–22
alcohol
　bone density and, 25, 30, 38, 262
　moderate, and increase in estrogen, 43
　osteoporosis and, 43–44, 244, 245
alendronate (Fosamax), xii, 193, 200, 201,
　203–7, 219
　for men, 247
　for steroid-induced osteoporosis, 259
anabolic steroids (androgenic steroids),
　226–27
anorexia nervosa, 46, 47, 251–52
autoimmune disease (lupus, asthma, copd,
　or inflammatory bowel disease)
　bone loss and, 30–31
　osteoporosis risk and, 109

back
　bone scans and MRI,137–38, 140
　chronic pain, 14, 16

compression fractures, 14, *15,* 136, 137,
　138
dowager's hump (exaggerated kyphosis),
　14–15, 107
height loss, 15–16
types of vertebral fractures, *15*
vertebral column, *13*
vertebral fractures, 12, 14–18, *13, 15,
　18,* 21, 106, 136
See also height loss
beta carotene, 95–96
blood tests, 129
　for bone turnover (n-telopeptide [NTX]
　　or c-telopeptide [CTX]), 133–35, 139,
　　240
　cortisol levels, for pituitary tumor or
　　Cushing's syndrome, 131–32
　monitoring treatment and, 237, 240
　for multiple myeloma (protein
　　electrophotesis), 131
　parathyroid level, 130
　transglutaminase antibodies, for celiac
　　disease (gluten-sensitive enteropathy),
　　131, 140
　tryptase, for mastocytosis, 132, 140
　vitamin D deficiency or insufficiency,
　　130–31, 140
bone
　age and strength, 31

bone (*cont.*)
    blood and urine testing, 129–40
    body weight and density, 108
    cancellous or "spongy," *29,* 187
    coritical (compact), 187
    discrepancies between one skeletal site
        and another, 127
    disease and accelerated loss, 30–31
    family history and genetics, importance
        of, 5, 7, 38
    gender, race, genetics and density or
        osteoporosis prevalence, 24, 126
    hormones and, 25–26
    lifestyle factors and density, 25
    loss, causes of, 25, 26–31, *28, 29,* 30–31,
        72–73
    menopause and, 27, 28–29, 110
    modeling, 26–27, 28
    osteoblasts, 27, 29, 228, 231
    osteoclasts, 27, 194, 211–12, 231
    osteocyte, 257
    peak bone mass, 22, *23,* 23–25, 26, 38,
        73, 104
    quality, 31, 109–10
    trabeculae, 27–28, 31
    turnover levels, 6, 133–35
    See also calcium
bone biopsy, 129, 138–39
bone density screening, 112–22
    age and, Caucasian women sixty-five and
        older, 104–5, 111
    central dual X-ray absorptiometry
        (DXA), 112–15, 116, 117, 118, 127,
        263
    future research and, 263
    genetic predisposition to low mass and,
        38
    hand radiographs, 118–19
    fractures and, 17
    hip bone mineral density (BMD), 114,
        115, 116, 118, 121, 122, 138
    men, 245–46
    menopausal and postmenopausal, 8, 105,
        109, 111, 260
    monitoring treatment and, 236, 238, 240
    peripheral DXA and SXA (single X-ray
        absorptiometry), 115–17, 128
    premenopausal women, 7–8, 249–50

quantitative computed tomography
    (QCT), 118
    T-Score, 119–20, *122,* 126, 128, 263
    ultrasound, 117–18
    Z-Score, 120–22, *122,* 126, 128
bone scans and MRI,137–38, 140
boron, 90
Breast Cancer Prevention Trial (BCPT),
    184

calcitonin (Miacalcin), xii, 162, 193–99
calcitriol, 227–28
calcium, 49–70
    bone density and, 25, 30
    childhood, 50–51
    dietary influences of other nutrients (salt,
        protein, phosphates), 52–53, 70
    dietary recommendations, fitting calcium
        into, 59–60
    estimating dietary calcium, 60–62, *61*
    excess, problems with, 65–66
    food labels, reading for calcium content,
        59
    food sources, 53, *54–55,* 55–56
    fortified foods, 56–57, *58, 59*
    lactose intolerance and, 66–67
    loss, daily, 50
    magnesium and, 91–92
    malabsorption syndromes and, 67–68, 92
    recommended intake, 50–52, *51*
    recommended intake, adjusting for
        malabsorption, 68
    skeleton composition and, 89
    supplements, 62–66, 70, 200, 245, 259,
        261
    supplements and constipation, 92
    vitamin D and, 68–70
celiac disease (gluten-sensitive enteropathy),
    131
    blood test for transglutaminase
        antibodies, 131, 140
constipation
    calcium supplements and, 92
    fracture and, 17, 146
copper, 90
corticosteroids. *See* steroids
Cushing's syndrome, 131–32, 140

diabetes, bone loss and, 25

diuretics, thiazide-containing, 132, 233
dowager's hump (exaggerated kyphosis),
14–15, 107

estrogen, 166
   alcohol and increased, 43–44
   bone density and, 25, 105, 166–67
   drop in, menopause, and bone loss, 105,
      110
   phytoestrogens for, 93–94
   smoking and, 40
   See also hormone or estrogen therapies
etidronate, 209–10
Evista (raloxifene), xii, 162, 163, 182,
   186–91
exercise, 6, 72–88, 201
   back muscles, strengthening, 80, *80, 81*
   bone density and, 30
   continuing, importance of, 77
   excessive, reduced bone mass and, 46–47,
      252
   facts, important, 83–84
   fall and fracture prevention, 73–74
   home program, 87–88
   muscle strengthening, 79–83, 85–87
   Pilates, 82, 201
   for steroid-induced osteoporosis, 261
   Tai Chi, 82
   therapeutic exercise program, after a
      fracture, 155–56
   tips for management of osteoporosis,
      84–88
   vertebral fractures, recommendations for
      sufferers of, 77–79
   weight-bearing aerobic, 75–76, 85
   weight control and, 74
   yoga, 82–83

falls
   chronic diseases and, 109
   dowager's hump (exaggerated kyphosis)
      and, 14–15
   exercise and prevention, 74
   medications and risk, 32, 44–45
   in men, 244
   reducing risk, 44–46, 154–55
   risk factors, 32–33
family history of osteoporosis. *See* genetic
   risk

FIT (Fracture Intervention Trial), 204, 205
fluoride, 228–29
Forteo, 162, 193, 239, 247. *See also*
   parathyroid hormone (PTH or Forteo)
Fosamax (alendronate), xii, 193, 201,
   203–7, 247, 248
fracture, 11
   adult, with little trauma, 106–7, 151,
      157
   back spasms with, 145
   compression, 14, *15,* 136, 137, 138, 146
   exercise and prevention, 74
   exercise recommendations for sufferers of
      vertebral, 77–79
   falls and, 15, 20–21
   family history of osteoporosis-related,
      107–8
   forearm, 145
   gender and, 21
   hip, 18–19, 40–41, 95, 106, 144,
      170–71, 221–22, 231, 243, 248
   increasing occurrence, 12
   instant morphometric or lateral vertebral
      imaging, 137
   lack of symptoms, 14
   low bone density and risk, 125
   muscle spasms with, 146
   neck, 20
   pelvic, 20
   race, ethnicity and, 21, 26
   rib, 20, 135–36, 145
   shoulder or proximal humerous, 144–45
   smoking and, 40–41
   spontaneous, 14, 21
   steroid use and increased risk, 258
   thyroid hormone and, 41–42
   vertebral, 12, *13,* 14–18, *15, 18,* 21,
      106, 136, 145–48
   vitamin D and prevention, 69
   wrist, 12, 20, 145
   X rays for, 135–37, 139–40, 143, 144
fracture care and rehabilitation, 143–57
   back braces, 147–48
   fall prevention, 154–55, 157
   hip replacement, 144
   orthopedist for, 156
   outpatient physical therapy, 146–47
   pain relief, 146
   physical therapy, 147, 148, 157

fracture care and rehabilitation (*cont.*)
  rehabilitation programs, 151–52
  safety concepts for the back, 152–54
  support groups, 156, 157
  surgery for distal leg fractures, 144
  therapeutic exercise program, 155–56,
    157
  vertebral fractures, 145–48, 150, 156–57
  vertebroplasty/kyphoplasty procedures,
    149–51

genetic risk
  bone density tests and, 38
  family history of osteoporosis-related
    fractures, 107–8, 110
  importance of, 38
  low bone mass and, 5, 7, 23–24
  medical history of parents and
    grandparents, 5, 26, 107
glucocorticoids and GCIOP
  (glucocorticoid-induced osteoporosis).
  See steroids
growth hormone agents, 230–31

height loss, 14, 15–16, 21
  abdominal distension and, 17, 21
  chronic digestive symptoms and, 17
  conditions other than osteoporosis and,
    107–8
  constipation and, 17
  monitoring treatment for osteoporosis
    and, 235–36, 239
  osteoporosis risk and, 107–8
  reduction of lower thorax or upper
    abdomen, and chronic pain, 16
  shortness of breath and restricted
    breathing, 15–16, 21
  X rays to determine cause, 126, 139–40
HIP (Hip Intervention Program), 208
hip fracture, 18–19, 95, 106
  death and, 19, 21
  falls and, 18
  hormone therapy and, 170–71
  lack of mobility and independence
    following, 19, 21
  in men, 243, 247
  mental decline, 19
  replacement, 144
  surgical repair, 19

HERS trial, 171, 173
hormone or estrogen therapies, 162, 163,
    165–81
  cancer decrease, 176
  cancer risk, 175–76
  effects of, various, 177
  estrogen administration, 171–72
  estrogen plus progestin vs. placebo, *179*
  estrogens, progestins and combination
    products, *167–68*
  progestin administration, 171–72
  reactions to the WHI news, 178–79
  remaining questions about, 177–78
  skeletal effects, 168–71
  vascular disease and, 172–74
hypothyroidism, 42–43

ipriflavone, 94–95, 99

juvenile kyphosis, 108

kidney stones, excess calcium and, 66, 132,
    140, 233

lactose intolerance, 66–67
lifestyle, sedentary, 38, 72–75. *See also*
    exercise; nutrition

magnesium, 91–92
malabsorption syndromes
  calcium and, 67–68, 92
  vitamin K deficiency and, 97–98, 99
manganese, 90–91
mastocytosis, 132, 139, 140
medications causing bone loss, 41–43, 110
  antiseizure medications, 43
  chemotherapy and, 43
  immunosuppressive drugs, 43
  osteoporosis risk and, 109
  steroids (glucocorticoid or
    corticosteroids), 25, 31, 41–42, 48,
    256–62
  thyroid hormone, 42–43
medications and falling risk, 32, 44–45
medications for osteoporosis
  alendronate (Fosamax), xii, 193, 200,
    201, 203–7, 219, 247, 248, 259
  anabolic steroids (androgenic steroids),
    226–27

bisphosphonates (alendronate, risedronate, etidronate, tiludronate, clodronate, pamidronate, zoledronic acid), 200–213
calcitriol, 227–28
etidronate, 209–10
fluoride, 228–29
growth hormone agents, 230–31
hormone or estrogen therapies, 162, 163, 165–81
monitoring treatment, 235–40
nasal calcitonin (Miacalcin), xii, 162, 193–99
nitrates, 231
Nolvadex, 183
pamidronate, 210
parathyroid hormone (PTH or Forteo), xii, 6, 104, 162, 193, 194, 214–25, *218*, 239, 247
raloxifene (Evista), xii, 162, 163, 182, 186–91
risedronate (Actonel), xii, 193, 207–9, 219, 259–60
SERMS (Selective Estrogen Receptor Modulators), 163, 182–92
statins, 231–32
strontium ranelate, 232
tamoxifen, 163, 182, 183–86, 191
thiazides, 132, 233
tibolone, 233–34
who should take, 158–62, 164
zoledronic acid, 211, 213, 264
medications for pain, 146, 199. *See also* pain
men, 243–49
alendrontate for, 247, 248
bone density testing and, 104, 245
bone mass and, 24
calcium intake daily, 247
calcium supplements, 245
diseases contributing to osteoporosis in, 244
falling risk, 244
hip fracture in, 243, 247
PHT (Forteo, Teriparatide), 247, 248
prevention in, 244–45
prevalence in, 243
prostate cancer and osteoporosis, 244
risk factors, 243–44

testosterone decline and bone loss, 25–26, 110, 244
testosterone therapy, 227
vertebral fractures in, 246–47
vitamin D intake daily, 247
vitamin D supplements, 245
menopause
accelerated bone loss, 30, 110
bone density screening, 8, 105, 109
bone loss and, 27, 28–29, 30
bone turnover and, 133
osteopenia and, 122–24, *123*
osteoporosis, prevalence, *123*
phytoestrogens for, 93–94
undiagnosed low BMD in, *125*
menstruation, 25, 46–47, 48, 251, 252
methotrexate, 43
Miacalcin (calciton), xii, 162, 193–99
MORE (Multiple Outcomes of Raloxifene Evaluation), 186, 188, 189, 190
multiple myeloma, blood test for (protein electrophotesis), 131

National Osteoporosis Foundation, 156
neck
dowager's hump (exaggerated kyphosis), 14–15
fracture, 20
pain, 14–15
New York State Osteoporosis Prevention and Education Programs, 156
NHANES (National Health and Nutrition Education Survey), 204–5
nitrates, 231
Novartis. *See* calcitonin
Nurses Health Study, 95
nutrition
calcium, 49–68, *54–55*
calcium-fortified foods, 56–57, *58*
canned fish with bones, 53, *55*
dairy foods, *54,* 55–56
dietary recommendations, fitting calcium into, 59–60
five servings of fruits and vegetables a day, 98
food labels, reading for calcium content, 59
foods that decrease calcium absorption, 52

nutrition (*cont.*)
    omega-3 fatty acids, 92–93
    phytoestrogens, 93–94
    prevention and, 39
    protein consumption, 52–53
    salt intake, 52–53
    soda intake (phosphates), 53
    soy products, *58*
    summary, 70–71
    vegetables, 53, *55*
    vitamin D, 68–70
    See also calcium

omega-3 fatty acids, 92–93
oral contraceptives, 6–7, 47
osteoarthritis, 11–12
osteopenia, 120, 122–26, *123*
    undiagnosed low BMD in
        postmenopausal women, *125*
osteopetrosis, 31
osteoporosis
    bone with, *30*
    bone remodeling cycle and bone loss, *28*
    consequences, *18*
    future research and treatments, 263–64
    prevalence data, 12, 121–22, *123*
    risk factors, 103–11
    what it is, 9–12
    See also bone; fractures; genetic risk;
        medications for osteoporosis;
        menopause; *specific topics*

pain
    chronic back, 11, 14, 16, 17
    controlling, 16
    flank area, 16, 21
    fractures, 17
    medication, 146, 199
    muscle spasms and, 146
    neck, 14
    vertebroplasty/kyphoplasty for vertebral
        fractures, 149–51
    X rays for cause, 135–37, 139–40, 143
Pamidronate, 210
parathyroid, 215
    blood test for hyperparathyroidism, 130,
        140
    hyperparathyroidism, 215–16
    tumor and, 130

parathyroid hormone (PTH or Forteo), xii,
    6, 104, 162, 193, 194, 214–25, *218*
    frequently asked questions, 221–25
    for men, 247, 248
phytoestrogens, 93–94, 99
premenopausal women, 249–55
    anorexia nervosa, 46, 47, 251–52
    bone density screening, 7–8, 249–50,
        254–55
    bone health steps for, 254
    bulemia and osteoporosis in, 252
    diseases and bone loss, 253–54, 255
    endometriosis and bone loss, 252–53
    exercise, excessive and lack of
        menstruation, 46–47, 252
    low bone density in, 3–6, 125–26
    menstruation irregularity, 255
    pituitary gland or hypothalmus tumors
        and bone loss, 253
    premature ovarian failure and, 253
    steroid treatment and, 255
    transient osteoporosis, 250–51, 254
prevention, 7, 37–38
    alcohol use, 43–44
    medications causing bone loss, 41–43
    in men, 244–45
    menstruation, keeping normal, 46–47,
        48
    nutrition, 49–71
    reducing falling risk, 44–46
    smoking, 40–41
    summary, 47–48
    See also exercise; nutrition
PROOF study (Prevention of Recurrence of
    Osteoporotic Fractures), 196–98

radiology procedures, 129
rheumatoid arthritis
    bone density and, 25
    osteoporosis risk and, 109
risedronate (Actonel), xii, 193, 207–9, 219
    steroid-induced osteoporosis, 259–60
risedronate clinical trial, 120
risk factors, 103–11
    adult fractures with little trauma, 106–7
    age, 104–6
    body weight, 108, 110
    bone quality, 109–10

chronic diseases, 109, 110, 244, 253–54, 255
genetics, 107–8, 110
height loss, 107–8
in men, 243–44
menopause, 27, 28–29, 30, 110
other, 109
race or ethnicity, 110, 124
smoking, 108–9, 110
steroids, 25, 31, 41–42, 48, 256–62
testosterone decline, 25–26, 110, 244
RUTH (Raloxifene Use in the Heart), 190

Scheurmann's disease, 107
SERMS (Selective Estrogen Receptor Modulators), 163, 182–92
raloxifene (Evista), xii, 162, 163, 182, 186–91
tamoxifen, 163, 182, 183–86, 191
smoking
bone density and, 25, 30, 38
estrogen reduction and, 40
hip fracture and, 40–41
osteoporosis risk and, 108–9, 262
prevention of osteoporosis and, 40–41
soy products, *58*, 93–94
STAR (Study of Tamoxifen and Raloxifene), 189
statins, 231–32
steroids (glucocorticoid or corticosteroids), 25, 31, 41–42, 48, 256–62
calcium supplements, 259, 261
exercise, 261
medications for osteoporosis, 259–61
smoking, drinking cessation and, 262
vitamin D supplements, 259, 261
strontium ranelate, 232
supplements
calcium, 62–66, 70, 92, 200, 259, 261
ipriflavone warning, 94–95, 99
magnesium, 92
multivitamin, 71, 98
multivitamin with folic acid, 96
vitamin D, 69, 200, 259, 261
vitamin K, 97
support groups, 156
symptoms
deformity, 11, 14–15, 21
disability, 11, 19

fractures, 11, 12, 14–18, *15, 18*
lack of, 7, 11, 14
pain, 11, 21

testosterone
decline and bone loss, 25–26, 110, 244
therapy, 227
thiazides, 132, 233
thyroid hormone
bone loss and, 42–43
hyperthyroidism, 140
TSH level tests, importance of, 47
tibolone, 233–34
Teriparatide, 247, 248
Turner's syndrome, 47

urine tests, 129
for bone turnover (pyridinium crosslinks), 133–35
calicum levels, 132, 233
cortisol levels, for pituitary tumor or Cushing's syndrome, 131–32, 140
excess calcium, 132, 140
monitoring treatment and, 237

VERT (Vertebral Fracture Studies), 207
vertebroplasty/kyphoplasty procedures, 149–51
vitamin A, 95–96
hip fracture increase and, 95
retinol, 95–96
vitamin B (folic acid, B12, B6), 96
vitamin C, 97
vitamin D
blood test for deficiency or insufficiency, 130–31, 140
calcitriol, 227–28
calcium absorption and, 68
dietary sources, 68
recommended doses for supplements, 69, 70, 71, 200, 245, 259, 261
sunlight and, 69
vitamin K, 97–98
vitamins, 80, 95–98. *See also specific vitamins;* supplements

weight, low
menstrual cessation, 46–47
osteoporosis risk and, 108, 110

women
  bone density, 24
  bone density, gender and race, 126
  bone density testing, 103–4
  estrogen and bone mass, 25
  fractures, race, ethnicity and, 21, 26
  menopausal, postmenopausal, bone
    density screening, 8, 105, 109, 260
  menopause and bone loss, 27, 28–29, 30,
    110
  menstruation and bone mass, 25, 46–47,
    48
  peak bone mass, *23*, 23–25
  premenopausal, bone density screening,
    7–8, 249–50
  premenopausal, low bone density in,
    3–6, 125–26, 249–55
  undiagnosed low BMD in
    postmenopausal women, *125*
Women's Health Initiative (WHI), 91–92,
    170–71, 174, 176, 177, 178–79, 180

X rays, 135–37, 139–40, 143, 144

  monitoring treatment and, 236, 239

zinc, 98
zoledronic acid, 211, 213, 264

Also Available from Warner Books

What Your Doctor May *Not* Tell You about Menopause

The Breakthrough Book on Natural Progesterone
by John R. Lee, M.D., with Virginia Hopkins

Most women experience hormone-related problems as they age and must consider synthetic hormone replacement therapy. But there is revolutionary news about completely safe, *natural progesterone*, the only hormone supplement older women may need. In this innovative book, Dr. Lee presents lifesaving facts that *even your doctor may not know*. He tells you how to stay energized, strong, and sexually vigorous, before menopause, during the menopausal years, and beyond.

"John Lee has pioneered work in women's health that has greatly influenced and enhanced the way I practice medicine."

—Christiane Northrup, M.D., author of
The Wisdom of Menopause

What Your Doctor May *Not* Tell You about Fibroids

New Techniques and Therapies—Including Breakthrough Alternatives to Hysterectomy

by Scott C. Goodwin, M.D., Michael Broder, M.D., and David Drum

Fibroids are benign tumors in the uterus that can grow large enough to cause bleeding, pain, or infertility. They are the leading reason for over 300,000 hysterectomies

more . . .

performed each year. Now Drs. Scott C. Goodwin and Michael Broder explore *all* the lifestyle strategies, medical therapies, and less invasive forms of surgery that may be able to control fibroids *without* a hysterectomy. This book will help you make the choice that's right for you.

What Your Doctor May *Not* Tell You About Autoimmune Disorders

The Revolutionary Drug-free Treatments for Thyroid Disease, Lupus, MS, IBD, Chronic Fatigue, Rheumatoid Arthritis, and Other Diseases

by Stephen B. Edelson, M.D., and Deborah Mitchell

An astonishing forty million Americans suffer from many forms of autoimmune diseases. Since these disorders are difficult to diagnose, most doctors simply treat each symptom separately, often leaving sufferers mistreated. Now a pioneering specialist has made a stunning connection between environmental toxins and all autoimmune disorders and developed an integrated treatment approach that will help you achieve lasting, healing results. Learn how to protect yourself from these diseases.